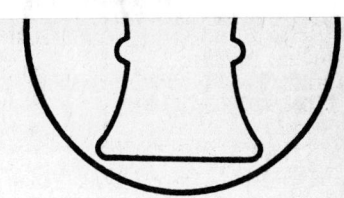

The Pharmacy Technician

MARVIN M. STOOGENKE, *B.S.*, *R.Ph.*

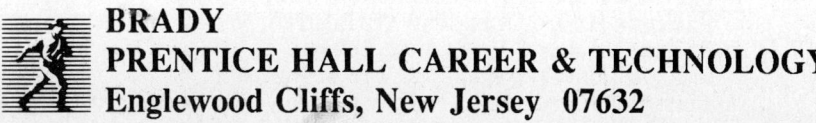

BRADY
PRENTICE HALL CAREER & TECHNOLOGY
Englewood Cliffs, New Jersey 07632

Library of Congress Cataloging-in-Publication Data

Stoogenke, Marvin M.
 The pharmacy technician.

 "A Brady book."
 Includes index.
 1. Pharmacy technicians. 2. Pharmacy. I. Title.
 [DNLM: 1. Pharmacists' Aids. 2. Pharmacy.
 QV 704 S882p]
 RS122.95.S76 1989   615'.4   88-17952
 ISBN 0-89303-799-0

Editorial/production supervision
and interior design: *Jane Bonnell*
Cover design: *20/20 Services, Inc.*
Manufacturing buyer: *Robert Anderson*

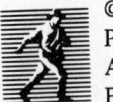

©1989 by Prentice Hall Career & Technology
Prentice-Hall, Inc.
A Paramount Communications Company
Englewood Cliffs, New Jersey 07632

All rights reserved. No part of this book may be
reproduced, in any form or by any means,
without permission in writing from the publisher.

Printed in the United States of America

10 9 8 7 6 5

ISBN 0-89303-799-0

PRENTICE-HALL INTERNATIONAL (UK) LIMITED, *London*
PRENTICE-HALL OF AUSTRALIA, PTY. LIMITED, *Sydney*
PRENTICE-HALL CANADA INC., *Toronto*
PRENTICE-HALL HISPANOAMERICANA, S.A., *Mexico*
PRENTICE-HALL OF INDIA PRIVATE LIMITED, *New Delhi*
PRENTICE-HALL OF JAPAN, INC., *Tokyo*
SIMON & SCHUSTER ASIA PTE., LTD., *Singapore*
EDITORA PRENTICE-HALL DO BRASIL, LTDA., *Rio de Janeiro*

To Judy, my confidante and critic,
who held a lighted candle at the end of the tunnel.
Her inspiration was the greatest part of my motivation.

To Scott, my computer expert and typist,
who devoted many hours of his college vacation to my project.
His conscientiousness assured the timeliness of this text.

To Jason, my artist,
who advised me of text aesthetics and provided me with an illustration.

To Saul,
who sacrificed many hours of playing time while I worked on this project.

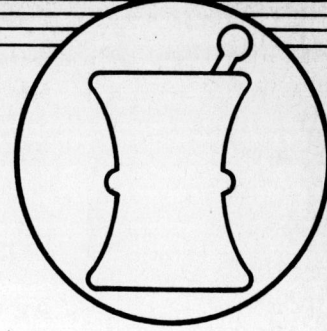

Contents

Preface ix

Trademark Acknowledgments xi

Introduction 1

1 Pharmacy Technology and the Study of Drug Monographs 3

The Status of Pharmacy Practice 3
The Role of Pharmacy Technicians 4
Reviewing Drug Monographs 6
Signs, Symptoms, and Side Effects 11

2 The Drug Order 15

The Script 16
The Physician's Order 23
Common Pharmaceutical Notations 25

3 Medical Terminology 34

Word Development: Usage and Components 34

4 Basics of Human Functioning 43

An Overview of Human Anatomy and Physiology 43
An Overview of Anatomical Systems 46

5 Arithmetic Review 72

Decimals 73
Percentage 78
Ratio and Proportion 84

6 Pharmacy Computations 87

Systems of Measure 87
The Apothecaries' System 89
The Metric System 90

7 Drug Classes 98

Analgesic 99
Antidiarrheal 100
Antihistamine 100
Anti-Infective 101
Antineoplastic 103
Antiulcer 105
Cardiovascular 105
Diuretic 107
Hormone 107
Laxative 108
Psychotherapeutic 109
Hypotensive 110
Anti-Inflammatory 111
Antigout 112
Muscle Relaxant 112
Bronchodilator 113
Supplement 113

Anticonvulsant 114
Antiarthritic 114
Ophthalmic 115
Hypoglycemic 117
Antinauseant/Antiemetic 117
Blood Modifier 118
Antispasmodic 118
AntiParkinson 119
Antitussive 119
Otic 120
Dermatologic 120
Vaginal 122
Antiobesity 123

8 Intravenous Pharmacy 124

History of Intravenous Therapy 124
Advantages and Disadvantages 125
Anatomy and Physiology of Intravenous Therapy 127
Tools of the Trade 130
Intravenous Calculations 136
Calculations Practice 140

Appendix A	Trade and Generic Names of Common Drugs	147
Appendix B	Common Drug Interactions	152
Appendix C	Practice Prescriptions	156
Appendix D	Practice Hospital Orders	176
Appendix E	Common Laboratory Tests	191
Appendix F	Commonly Used Diluents	194
Appendix G	Common Vitamin Names	195

Appendix H	Drugs New and Coming Through	196
	Glossary	198
	Index	203

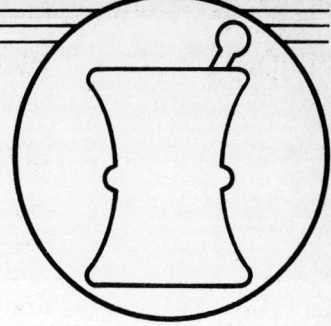

Preface

This text is your key to a formidable and fulfilling career as a pharmacy technician. As a pharmacy technician you will become an integral part of the allied health team composed of nurses, physician assistants, medical technologists, physical therapists, and other paraprofessionals who are committed to the safety, care, and well-being of the patient.

Pharmacy services have expanded and grown at an accelerated rate, paving a new way for pharmacy technicians. We cannot overemphasize the significance pharmacy technicians have upon pharmacy operations and the substantial part they play in the health care work force. As pharmacy services continue to grow, with new services being offered, new drugs entering the market, and comprehensive drug information becoming a necessity, the need for pharmacy technicians increases.

Many of the traditional pharmacy functions, once performed by pharmacists, are now being performed by pharmacy technicians as pharmacists pursue new and expanded roles. The pharmacy technician has assumed a position which supports and enhances the progressive direction taken by pharmacy. The pharmacy technician has become the key person in assuring the smooth and uninterrupted functioning of traditional pharmacy services.

The field of pharmacy technology will provide you with stimulating work and positive growth potential in hospitals, clinics, skilled nursing facilities, retail pharmacies, health maintenance organizations, and the armed services. As a pharmacy technician you will be engaged in the dispensing and prepackaging of medications, drug compounding, intravenous preparations, and various other facets in an active and progressive pharmacy.

The demand and opportunities for pharmacy technicians are continuing to increase. Salaries have risen substantially, position availabilities and placement have increased, and the impact of pharmacy technology on the marketplace has impressed hospital administrators and pharmacy managers. The field of pharmacy technology is young and full of opportunities. As you enter this career you will become a vital part in the fascinating world of the health professional.

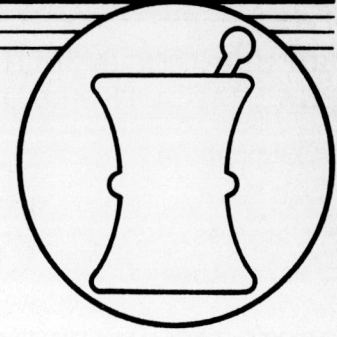

Trademark Acknowledgments

Each of the following drugs is a registered trademark of the company beneath which it is listed.

ABBOTT LABORATORIES

    E.E.S.
    Enduron
    Erythrocin
    K-Tab
    Liposyn
    Ogen
    Oretic
    Panwarfin
    Tranxene

ADRIA LABORATORIES

    Ilozyme
    Kaon

ALTO PHARMACEUTICALS, INC.

    Zinc-220

ARMOUR PHARMACEUTICAL COMPANY

    Thytropar

AYERST LABORATORIES

    Inderal
    Mysoline
    Premarin

BEACH PHARMACEUTICALS

    K-Phos

BEECHAM LABORATORIES

    Amoxil
    Beepen VK
    Larotid

BERLEX LABORATORIES, INC.

    Qinaglute Dura-Tabs

BOEHRINGER INGELHEIM PHARMACEUTICALS, INC.

- Alupent
- Atrovent
- Catapres
- Persantine

BOOTS PHARMACEUTICALS, INC.

- Lopurin
- Rufen

BRISTOL LABORATORIES

- K-Lyte
- Polycillin
- Polymox

BURROUGHS WELLCOME CO.

- Lanoxin
- Retrovir
- Septra
- Zovirax
- Zyloprim

CIBA PHARMACEUTICAL COMPANY

- Apresoline
- Esidrix
- Ludiomil
- PBZ[1]
- Ritalin
- Serpasil
- Slow-K
- Transderm-Nitro

DERMIK LABORATORIES, INC.

- Hytone
- Zetar

DISTA PRODUCTS COMPANY

- Ilosone
- Keflex
- Nalfon
- Nebcin

Du PONT PHARMACEUTICALS, INC.

- Coumadin
- Percocet

ELDER PHARMACEUTICALS, INC.

- Pabanol

FISONS CORPORATION

- Intal
- Kondremul

FLINT LABORATORIES, INC.

- Synthroid

FOREST PHARMACEUTICALS, INC.

- Kay Ciel

GEIGY PHARMACEUTICALS

- Brethine
- Lopressor
- Tegretol

GERIATRIC PHARMACEUTICAL CORP.

- Cevi-Bid

GLAXO, INC.

- Ventolin
- Zantac

HOECHST-ROUSSEL PHARMACEUTICALS, INC.

- Diabeta
- Festal
- Lasix
- Topicort
- Trental

---

[1] CIBA CONSUMER PHARMACEUTICALS

Trademark Acknowledgments

ICI PHARMA

Nolvadex
Sorbitrate
Tenormin[2]

JANSSEN PHARMACEUTICA INC.

Imodium
Monistat

KABIVITRUM, INC.

Intralipid

KEY PHARMACEUTICALS, INC.

Nitro-Dur
Theo-Dur

KNOLL PHARMACEUTICALS

Isoptin

LAKESIDE PHARMACEUTICALS

Bentyl
Nicorette

LEDERLE LABORATORIES

Achromycin V
Folvite
Ledercillin VK
Minocin
Neptazane

ELI LILLY and COMPANY

Betalin S
Ceclor
Darvocet-N
Darvon Compound
Dymelor
Hexa-Betalin
Humulin
V-Cillin K

LYPHOMED, INC.

Pentam 300

MARION LABORATORIES, INC.

Carafate
Cardizem
Ditropan
Nitro-Bid
Os-Cal

McGAW LABORATORIES

FreAmine
Hyperlyte R

McNEIL PHARMACEUTICAL

Haldol
Tolectin
Tylenol[3]

MEAD JOHNSON PHARMACEUTICALS

Colace
Desyrel
Duricef
Klotrix

MERCK SHARP & DOHME

Aldomet
Benemid
Blocadren
Clinoril
Cogentin
Diuril
Dolobid
Elavil
Flexeril
HydroDIURIL
Indocin
Mephyton

---

[2] STUART division of ICI
[3] McNEIL CONSUMER PRODUCTS CO.

Midamor
Mevacor
Noroxin
Timoptic
Vasotec

MERRELL DOW PHARMACEUTICALS, INC.

Metahydrin
Norpramin
Quinamm
Seldane

MILES INC. PHARMACEUTICAL DIVISION

Cipro
Stilphostrol

NORWICH EATON PHARMACEUTICALS, INC.

Macrodantin

ORGANON INC.

Cotazyme

ORTHO PHARMACEUTICAL CORPORATION

Ortho-Novum
Retin-A

PARKE-DAVIS[4]

Adrenalin
Aplisol
Benadryl
Centrax
Dilantin
ERYC
Lopid
Meclomen
Nitrostat

Pitocin
Procan SR

PENNWALT PRESCRIPTION DIVISION

Adapin
Zaroxolyn

PFIZER LABORATORIES DIVISION

Diabinese
Feldene
Minipress
Pfizerpen
Procardia
Renese
Vibramycin
Vibra-Tabs
Vistaril[5]

PRINCETON PHARMACEUTICAL PRODUCTS

Corgard
Naturetin

A.H. ROBINS COMPANY

Micro-K
Quinidex
Reglan
Robitussin
Viokase

ROCHE LABORATORIES

Bactrim
Bumex
Dalmane
Gantrisin
Larodopa
Librium
Synkavite
Valium

[4]*Note:* The Amcill brand of ampicillin manufactured by Parke-Davis is currently manufactured as the generic by its generics subsidiary, Warner-Chilcott.

[5]oral dosage form

Trademark Acknowledgments

ROERIG
- Atarax
- Glucotrol
- Navane
- Sinequan
- Vistaril[6]

RORER PHARMACEUTICALS
- Hygroton
- Levothroid
- Lozol
- Maalox
- Slo-Bid
- Slo-Phyllin

SANDOZ PHARMACEUTICALS CORPORATION
- D.H.E. 45
- Hydergine
- Mellaril
- Restoril
- Tavist
- Visken

SCHERING CORPORATION
- Chlor-Trimeton
- Garamycin
- Lotrimin
- Normodyne
- Proventil
- Trinalin
- Valisone
- Vanceril

SEARLE PHARMACEUTICALS INC.
- Aldactone
- Calan
- Flagyl
- Norpace

SMITH KLINE & FRENCH LABORATORIES
- Compazine
- Dyazide
- Dyrenium
- Ecotrin[7]
- Eskalith
- Feosol[7]
- Tagamet

E.R. SQUIBB & SONS INC.
- Capoten
- Pentids
- Principen
- Rubramin PC[8]
- Sumycin
- Veetids

SYNTEX LABORATORIES, INC.
- Anaprox[9]
- Lidex
- Naprosyn[9]
- Nasalide

THE UPJOHN COMPANY
- Cleocin
- Cortef
- Deltasone
- E-Mycin
- Halcion
- Medrol
- Micronase
- Motrin
- Orinase
- Provera
- Solu-Medrol
- Tolinase
- Xanax

[6] parenteral dosage form
[7] SMITHKLINE CONSUMER PRODUCTS
[8] SQUIBB-MARSAM, INC.
[9] SYNTEX PUERTO RICO, INC.

USV LABORATORIES, INC.

Thyrar

WARNER-LAMBERT

Lubriderm

WESTWOOD PHARMACEUTICALS, INC.

Keralyt

WILLEN DRUG COMPANY

Neutra-Phos

WINTHROP PHARMACEUTICALS

Demerol
Hypaque
Luminal
Talwin NX

WYETH LABORATORIES

Amphogel
Ativan
Isordil
Omnipen
Pen Vee K
Phenergan
Serax
Wycillin
Wymox
Wytensin

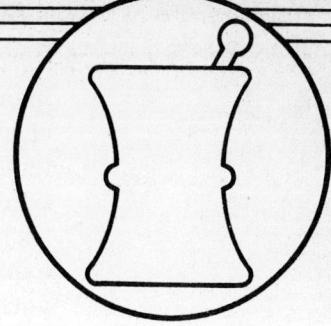

Introduction

Acquisition of this text is an indication of your interest in being a pharmacy technician and of your desire to competently perform those activities associated with pharmacy technology. This text offers you the opportunity to examine and pursue a career as a pharmacy technician, by providing you with the means necessary to enter the field of pharmacy technology.

Pharmacy technology deals with the practical everyday medication needs of the patient. The content of this text is derived from actual prescriptions and hospital Physician's Orders. Each skill area has been elaborated upon to provide a basic understanding of pharmacy knowledge which can be applied in every pharmacy environment.

The role of the pharmacy technician requires a battery of basic skills as well as the knowledge to perform pharmacy procedures effectively. These procedures ultimately encompass the preparation and distribution of drugs. This text thoroughly discusses the components of these procedures, which comprise the traditional practice of pharmacy.

As you study each chapter, you will learn how to practice each aspect of pharmacy being discussed. The initial chapters introduce the role of the pharmacy technician, pharmacy terminology, and important abbreviations. They discuss drug monographs and prescription screening and review hospital Physician's Orders for medication. The necessary components of the prescription are examined, with particular emphasis on common errors made by prescribers. Finally, they deal with the requirements necessary to dispense the medication properly, which include proper labeling, additional information labels for specific situations, and appropriate containers for special drugs.

Subsequent chapters discuss calculating dosages, weights and measures, and conversions. Weights and measures are the rudiments of pharmacy. Knowledge of measures must be explicit in order to perform the conversions required for compounding or calculating quantities for the patient as directed by the physician. The text reviews ratio and proportion, which is the relationship of quantities of drugs, expressed as a part of the total medication. In the calculations chapter you will learn to solve problems and convert from one type of measure to another. The calculations chapter is designed to give you the needed tools and methodology which will ultimately make you comfortable with their use, and competent in their use.

Metrology, which is the term used in pharmacy for measures, calculations, and conversions as an aggregate study, is followed by a study in drugs. The aim of the drug chapters (and corresponding appendices) is to provide you with an enumeration of drug classes, their intended uses, common trade and generic names of representative drugs on the market, and to introduce you to general common drug side effects and interactions.

The remaining chapters consider a number of other pharmacy-related areas, including anatomy, physiology, medical terminology, and intravenous admixtures. Appendices containing prescriptions and hospital Physician's Orders are provided for reference and practice.

This text presents basic pharmacy knowledge ready to be applied. Each chapter provides a structured learning process that is designed to guide you through an array of information that will be enhanced by your actual on-the-job activities.

As with any career, your particular accomplishment as a pharmacy technician depends upon your personal commitment to pharmacy technology. The personal qualities you will need, in order to be properly oriented and prepared as a technician, begin with your degree of interest. This text will serve as a guide, and help transform your ability into capability.

Pharmacy Technology and the Study of Drug Monographs

The scope of this text is to present a basic instructional guide for learning the elements of pharmacy as it pertains to current pharmacy practice and to the pharmacy technician's role changes in the future. Therefore, rather than listing over 100 drugs, their uses, side effects, and interactions, this chapter provides a process for reviewing drugs. The format was designed to accommodate three criteria:

1. The review of drugs should be efficient and effective.
2. The review of drugs should be uniform.
3. The review should be expandable to provide for new drugs entering the marketplace.

Before we get to the drug literature review process, let's look at the status of pharmacy and how the role of the pharmacy technician has developed.

THE STATUS OF PHARMACY PRACTICE

There was a time when pharmacy was an art. The correct compounding process and the final elegance of the product was the state-of-the-art philosophy. Terms such as "secundum artem" (Latin, meaning "according to the art") and "pharmaceutically elegant" evolved during those bygone years.

Pharmacy is substantially changed today, and is a highly complex scientific field. Advancements in dispensing hardware (for example, parenteral and enteral pumps, drug delivery systems, counters, and dispensing systems) and the development of high-powered, potent drugs have created a reduced need for the art and a significantly increased need for knowing and understanding massive amounts of information required to assure the greatest possible safety and effective outcome of drug therapy for patients.

THE ROLE OF PHARMACY TECHNICIANS

Sophisticated advances in technology, changes in social attitudes about health, and concerns over health care economics have impacted on pharmacy in another way. Pharmacists who traditionally have provided drug dispensing services are now moving into new facets of pharmacy (for example, computer technology, high-risk drug monitoring, financial management, and specialized pharmacy such as outpatient parenteral chemotherapy and parenteral nutrition). The traditional pharmacy workload (filling drug orders and dispensing) is increasingly handled by pharmacy support staff. The pharmacy technician's expanding role will require more extensive expertise in the areas of drug dosages, side effects, predictable reactions, and other drug-related issues.

The pharmacy technician is the final link in the continuity of care between the patient and the illness, and the patient and the drug. The pharmacy technician supplies the drugs and the information, and, as the protector of a patient's health, must make every effort to assure that the patient's rights and expectations are met.

PATIENT'S RIGHTS OF EXPECTATION

The patient has the right to expect:

- protection from unwanted discomfort resulting from drug therapy
- information regarding side effects, drug reactions, and other drug-related limiting characteristics
- preparedness for both the expected and unexpected occurrences due to drug therapy
- vigilant efforts to assure reasonable safety in drug therapy
- professional service and pharmacy expertise with each drug dispensed
- complete, comprehendible, and current information on each drug dispensed
- maintenance of confidentiality

The patient has responsibilities also. These obligations, however, should be expected only after the pharmacy technician has met his or her obligations and presented the patient with appropriate instructions. At times, it may be necessary to remind patients of some of these responsibilities, in order to assure the greatest safety and best outcome for the chosen drug therapy.

PATIENT'S RESPONSIBILITIES

The patient is responsible for:

- providing complete and accurate information
- complying with given directions
- communicating unfavorable signs and symptoms after drug therapy has begun
- asking questions when instructions are not understood completely

Roles Change for Pharmacy Technicians

The pharmacy technician's role as a dispenser of medications is destined to grow. While it is unlikely that any pharmacy technician will be able to learn and retain all the facts about each drug, it is important that he or she provides the correct drug information in compliance with the patient's rights of expectation. The purpose of this chapter is to present a tool which will aid you in selecting facts which are pertinent to patients.

New Roles Require New Competencies

How does the pharmacy technician begin to learn the many facts about each drug? The keys to learning and remembering information are categorizing drug groups, aggregating consistent facts, and making some generalizations. Not all drugs are absolute and fall neatly into a class, category, or set of data. However, the pharmacy technician must screen for potential side effects, interactions, and other potentially limiting outcomes before the patient takes that first dose. The pharmacy technician must make the patient aware of potentially dangerous side effects. The patient must be urged to notify the physician when those signs or symptoms actually occur.

Confidence Builds on Competence

First, you must perform an academic exercise which will sharpen your curiosity and desire for probing. Learn to ask WHY? WHERE? and WHAT? After a while, you will become increasingly curious as the knowledge you acquire becomes filled with interest and surprises. As the information expands and the focused process for reviewing data permits you to retain large amounts of noteworthy information, your desire to probe further will sharpen.

Next, you must have an available source of authoritative references. These references include drug compendia, drug monographs, a medical dictionary, and a manual of illness and therapy.

REFERENCES

- Physicians' Desk Reference (PDR)
- American Hospital Formulary Service Drug Information

- AMA Drug Evaluations
- Compendium of Drug Therapy
- Dorland, Gould, or Taber Medical Dictionary
- The Merck Manual of Diagnosis and Therapy

(*Note:* These are only a few of the many available references.)

REVIEWING DRUG MONOGRAPHS

Finally, you need the instrument which will help you sort through thousands of pages of data and extract what is necessary for your needs: the drug monograph. Drug monographs have variable formats. Knowing what to review will save you enormous amounts of time. All manufacturer monographs provide the following information about each drug:

- description
- action — *how the drug works*
- indications
- contraindications
- usage in pregnancy
- adverse reactions
- dosages (and administration)
- packaging availability

Additional areas of information are available for drugs when the information is applicable. For instance, many applicable drug monographs may address the following areas:

- microbiology — *interference c̄ lab tests*
- warnings
- precautions
- laboratory interference
- drug abuse and dependency
- overdosage
- pharmacology (and toxicology)
- drug interactions

The Tool

The volume of information available for any drug is massive. It would be nice to learn and retain all the data that exists for each drug. However, the information you need to know about each drug in order to perform your job properly (that is, select the correct drug, guard patients against unnecessary harm and discomfort, and guide patients in taking drugs appropriately) can be reduced to a realistic workable knowledge of drugs. Whenever possible, try to review as much data about a drug as you can. Practically, however, time may not permit you to indulge in an intensive reading of the material. Therefore, you must focus your reading on the facts pertinent to your needs. The following format is a tool to extract important information. Consistency is also very important in your attempt to retain as much information as possible.

DRUG REVIEW FORMAT

1. generic drug name
2. representative drug trade name(s)
3. other identification
4. primary drug class
5. intended indications for use
6. other indications for use
7. dosage limits
8. potential drug and/or food interactions
9. potential unwanted drug effects
10. potential drug effect on existing disorders
11. potential drug interference on laboratory tests
12. noteworthy facts

1. Generic Drug Name. The generic name of the drug is the nonproprietary name. There is no legal protection that a manufacturer can obtain for a generic drug product. The implication is that any manufacturer can produce a generic product as long as there are no patented brand name drugs for a generic drug with a patent still in effect.

2. Representative Drug Trade Name(s). Trade names are also referred to as brand names. Manufacturers select these special drug names in order to protect their products under the United States patent laws, which enable the patent holder to be the sole source producer of the drug for the seventeen-year period during which a patent is in effect. For example, Inderal is the brand name for the generic drug propranolol. In addition, the generic drugs penicillin and phenoxymethyl penicillin have many brand names: Veetids, Pentids, Pen Vee K, Wycillin, V-Cillin K, and many more. (*Note:* Patent holders can license other manufacturers to produce a drug. Once a patent on a drug expires, any company can produce the drug under a new brand name and promote it, using that brand name.) Companies can produce the drug under its generic name also.

3. Other Identification. Some drugs are given acronyms or "nicknames." Many abbreviated names may be used universally, while others are used in a specific locale, hospital, or geographic section. For example, hydrochlorothiazide may also be written as HCTZ, chlortrimeton as CT, tetracycline as TCN, digoxin as dig, and nitroglycerin as TNG or NTG. (*Note:* E.E.S. is an acronym used by the manufacturer as their brand name product to represent erythromycin ethylsuccinate.)

4. Primary Drug Class. Some drugs may possess more than one clinical use. However, the drug will be categorized under a primary drug class. This class depends on the manufacturer's primary intended use and Food and Drug Administration (FDA) approval. Drugs are commonly found to have therapeutic use for multiple disorders. A prime example is propranolol. This drug was originally marketed as a beta-adrenergic blocking cardiovascular agent indicated for angina. Subsequently, propranolol was found to be effective in the treatment of migraine headaches. The drug is still primarily a cardiovascular agent, but its use for migraine headaches is widely accepted.

5. Intended Indications for Use. The disorders for which a drug is to be used are only identified after many years of research and clinical trials on patients. The drug producer submits a new drug application (NDA) to the FDA with an enormous amount of information to support the use and safety of the drug. Upon FDA approval, the manufacturer is able to market the drug for a particular indication.

6. Other Indications for Use. As you saw in item four, primary drug class, subsequent uses are often found for drugs. Consider the examples in Table 1-1.

TABLE 1-1
Multiple Uses of Drugs

Generic Drug	Intended Indication	Other Indications
acebutolol	hypertension	cardiac arrhythmias
atenolol	hypertension	angina
captopril	hypertension	heart failure (edema)
chlorthalidone	hypertension	edema
clorazepate	anxiety	epileptic seizures alcohol withdrawal

diazepam	anxiety	skeletal muscle
		   spasms
		   alcohol withdrawal

doxepin	depression	peptic ulcer
furosemide	edema	hypertension
nadolol	angina	hypertension
phenytoin	seizures	cardiac arrhythmias

7. Dosage Limits. The amount of a drug for each dose prescribed by the practitioner and taken by the patient represents the findings of many tests performed by drug producers, research institutions, universities, and individual practicing physicians. This dose is referred to as the *usual dose*. Often, dosages are variable to meet the needs of patients without harmful or annoying side effects. Dosage limits indicate the highest dose which can produce a desired therapeutic outcome without adverse effects. Dosage limits documented by drug manufacturers also refer to uncompromised patients (that is, patients without kidney, liver, or other disorders). Compromised patients require changes in dosages to compensate for their inability to metabolize a drug as in the uncompromised patient. These special drug requirements are addressed in the drug literature.

8. Potential Drug and Food Interactions. Generally, drug therapy and drug response is fairly unpredictable. Little has been documented in the area of food/drug interactions. The classic food/drug interaction case occurs in a class of drugs known as monoamine oxidase (MAO) inhibitors. MAO inhibitors are used primarily for the management of patients with depression. Hypertensive crisis has occurred in patients taking MAO inhibitors and ingesting foods in which aging or protein breakdown has been used to increase flavor. These foods include a variety of cheeses, sour cream, wine, beer, chicken liver, and more.

There has been considerable documentation regarding drug/drug interactions. These interactions are measured on their clinical significance (that is, what percent of the population taking the drug has experienced the interaction?). The documented impact of drug interactions on patients is an important benchmark, since many interactions may not be readily observable or measurably harmful for a majority of patients.

9. Potential Unwanted Drug Effects. You may be more familiar with this area referred to as drug side effects, adverse reactions, or untoward reactions. The word "unwanted" is stressed here because some side effects of drugs are desirable. For example, antihistamines are known for their sedative effect. Some companies have marketed sleeping compounds with an antihistamine as the active component.

Review the list at the end of this chapter for an understanding of the myriad of potentially unwanted drug effects. The list includes nearly every side effect which may occur from a drug therapy. These side effects were selected because they are observable by the patient and are, therefore, reportable. Changes in the quantity or quality of blood components have no value without a blood test. These changes are unobservable. However, unusual bruising is observable and may have significant meaning to the patient, physician, pharmacist, and the pharmacy technician.

10. Potential Drug Effects on Existing Disorders. You will not find many pharmacists reviewing prescribed drugs for their effect on existing disorders. The relationship between drugs and disorders is significant and should not be overlooked. The consumption of drugs known to affect an existing disorder may either mask the condition, thereby hiding the relevant signs requiring action, or exacerbate (worsen the condition of) the disorder. For example, ulcerative colitis may be worsened by the use of antibiotics such as amoxicillin, ampicillin, pencillin, and cefaclor, or by the use of nonsteroidal anti-inflammatory drugs such as ibuprofen and indomethacin.

11. Potential Drug Interference on Lab Tests. Drugs can have a marked effect on the results of blood, urine, and fecal laboratory tests. You should be aware of commonly performed tests, the range of normal measurement, and the drugs which can interfere with the test results.

Many of the following tests are performed routinely on patients:

> blood clotting tests
> complete blood count
> electrolyte tests
> erythrocyte sedimentation rates
> glucose tests
> heart enzyme tests
> kidney function tests
> lipid tests
> liver function tests
> occult blood tests
> routine urinalysis
> thyroid function tests
> uric acid test

An in-depth explanation of each test may be found in Appendix E.

12. Noteworthy Facts. Up to this point, you have followed a strict information-collecting format which permits little flexibility: review drug literature and check off the appropriate side effect, disorder, or laboratory test. But you should also jot down those bits of information often overlooked and never communicated to the patient. For instance:

1. A patient receiving drug therapy to treat hypertension should be reminded to comply with a low-salt diet requirement.
2. Patients being treated for genital herpes (apparent by the use of the antiviral drug, acyclovir) should be reminded that a threat exists of transmitting the virus while the lesions are visible.
3. The effects of allopurinol therapy for gout may first be noticeable between two and six weeks.
4. Superinfection is always a threat with prolonged use of antibiotic drug therapy.
5. Lactose is an inert ingredient in many preparations and should be noted for lactose intolerant patients.

These are just a few examples of noteworthy facts. As you proceed to review drugs and build your own reference on drugs, consider what patients have said to you regarding specific drugs. Jot this information down. Remember that all the idiosyncracies of a drug/person response are not contained in the literature, and nothing surpasses firsthand information based on actual experiences.

Review the following list of twenty-five popularly prescribed drugs. (This list was prepared to guide you with your first selection of drugs to review.)

Generic Name	Trade Name
1. triamterine/hydrochlorothiazide	DYAZIDE
2. acetaminophen/codeine	TYLENOL WITH CODEINE
3. propoxyphene/acetaminophen	DARVOCET-N
4. cimetidine	TAGAMET
5. atenolol	TENORMIN
6. ranitidine	ZANTAC
7. digoxin	LANOXIN
8. terfenadine	SELDANE
9. potassium chloride	SLOW K
10. phenytoin	DILANTIN
11. furosemide	LASIX
12. diazepam	VALIUM
13. nifedipine	PROCARDIA
14. amoxicillin	AMOXIL
15. conjugated estrogens	PREMARIN
16. ibuprofen	MOTRIN
17. piroxicam	FELDENE
18. alprazolam	XANAX
19. cephalexin	KEFLEX
20. metoprolol	LOPRESSOR
21. naproxen	NAPROSYN
22. erythromycin ethylsuccinate	E.E.S.
23. theophylline	THEO-DUR
24. cyclobenzaprine	FLEXERIL
25. norethindrone/ethinyl estradiol	ORTHO-NOVUM

Note: An expanded list may be found in Appendix A.

It is much easier to study and remember facts about drugs when you follow a consistent plan. Try to establish "rules of similarity" for drug classes. For example, drugs absorbed from the intestine such as long-acting or sustained release aspirin, all nonsteroidal anti-inflammatory agents, and beta-lactam antibiotics (for example, penicillins) should be monitored closely in patients with ulcerative colitis. Study drugs individually within the same drug group. For instance, study each drug in the antibiotic class or cardiac grouping. This method will highlight the similarities shared by each drug within the group.

SIGNS, SYMPTOMS, AND SIDE EFFECTS

Signs and Symptoms Tell Us Something

Many drug manufacturers perform studies to identify side effects which may occur while using a specific drug. Studies showing the incidence of side effects have not been abundant for many drugs. The subjectivity of many side effects such as drowsiness, cramps, thirst, and tingling presents a shortcoming in determining which side effects are truly significant. Even quantitative studies using blood, urine, and stool samples subjected to laboratory testing result in variable ranges of measurements.

Your role is instrumental because you are the last level of drug monitoring before the patient consumes the drug. You can be of substantive value to many patients by informing them of the high incidence of observable side effects of some drugs. Patients made aware of observable side effects are able to take timely action which may result in discomfort-free and harm-free drug therapy.

When a Side Effect Is Significant

There are few distinct guidelines, if any, to determine when a side effect is due to drug therapy or some other cause. Perhaps a general rule to adopt would be to answer the following questions: How much? How long? How unbearable?

"How much" refers to the quantity of the side effect. This situation can be illustrated nicely by using the common side effect of a rash. There are many types of rashes. The quantity or area affected will vary according to many patients. Quantity will depend on the area covered, the amount of itching or burning, the degree of redness, and other attributes of the rash. Other side effects may be quantified by the number of occurrences (for example, three sharp shooting pains over a four-hour period).

"How long" depends on the duration of the side effect. Some patients may not notice a side effect for a period of time. If, however, the degree of side effect makes the patient take notice, twenty-four to thirty-six hours should be ample allowable time to determine if the side effect is lessening. You can see how the quantity and duration may relate to each other.

Finally, a patient will certainly be aware of "how unbearable" or intense a side effect may be. A side effect may cover a large body area, occur often, or last for a period of time, but not be unbearable. For instance, a patient may be covered by a rash on a large area of his or her body and not experience any discomfort. The intensity supersedes "how much" and "how long," resulting in a phone call to the pharmacist or practitioner. Intensity is extremely important, as may be illustrated by severe rashes caused by gold-containing compounds used for arthritis. A physician may weigh the discomfort of the side effect against the benefit of the drug therapy in an effort to determine whether or not to continue with the drug.

You will often be asked questions concerning drug side effects. The most you can do is review the drug monograph for side effects. Then determine from the patient "how much," "how long," "how unbearable," before giving advice to the patient. Check with the pharmacist for concurrence.

Groupings of Side Effects Can Be Significant

Side effects alone may have little meaning. Groupings of side effects occurring during a period while a patient is on drug therapy may represent an entirely different story. The following groupings of side effects have been prepared to flag situations which require timely intervention. These combinations of signs and symptoms may be suggestive of severe unobservable events.

Signs, Symptoms, and Side Effects

SYMPTOMS OCCURRING DURING DRUG THERAPY REQUIRING IMMEDIATE NOTIFICATION OF PHYSICIAN

General Symptoms

- joint pain
- muscle pain
- fever
- chills
- unusual bleeding
- easy bruising
- sore throat
- sore mouth
- discolored tongue
- dark urine
- wheezing
- unusual/uncontrollable fatigue
- muscle weakness
- chest pain
- severe abdominal pain
- heart palpitations (pounding)
- excessive vomiting
- excessive diarrhea
- hallucinations
- depression
- yellowing skin

Specific Combinations of Symptoms

Superinfection (fungal overgrowth)
- black tongue
- hairy tongue
- sore tongue
- sore mouth
- glossitis

Serum Sickness
- chills
- fever
- arthralgia
- edema
- pruritus (itching)
- fatigue
- rash

Excessive Potassium Loss
- excessive thirst
- tiredness
- restlessness
- muscle pains/cramps
- nausea/vomiting
- increased or rapid heart rate/pulse

Jaundice
- yellowing skin
- yellowing eyeballs

Blood Component Changes
(*Note*: any combination of the following symptoms may represent a variety of blood changes or disorders such as agranulocytosis, leukopenia, beta-hemolytic anemia, or thrombocytopenia.)
- headache
- sore throat/sore mouth
- muscle weakness
- fatigue
- bruising
- unusual bleeding
- fever
- chills

Adverse Liver Involvement
- fever
- malaise
- right upper quadrant pain
- yellowing skin

Ulcerative Colitis
- diarrhea
- weight loss

Neuropathy
- numbness
- weakness
- incoordination

Fluid and Electrolyte Disturbances
- dry mouth
- thirst
- weakness
- lethargy
- drowsiness
- restlessness
- muscle pain/cramps
- muscle fatigue
- decreased urinary output
- irregular heartbeat/pulse

Sympathomimetic Nervous System Disturbances
- muscle cramps
- insomnia
- nausea
- weakness
- dizziness
- nervousness
- tremor
- headache
- tachycardia
- palpitations

Anticholinergic Responses
- blurred vision
- dry mouth
- mydriasis
- change in pulse rate
- drowsiness
- amnesia
- fatigue
- urinary retention
- constipation

Cholinergic Responses
- involuntary repetitive muscular movements
- nausea
- vomiting
- diarrhea
- miosis
- excessive salivation
- excessive sweating
- abdominal cramps
- bradycardia
- bronchospasm
- flushing
- lacrimation
- urinary urgency
- belching

Allergic Reaction
- urticaria (hives)
- pruritus
- clammy skin
- flushing
- acute bronchospasm
- shortness of breath
- fluid retention with swelling
- throat constriction
- cyanosis (blue coloring)
- wheezing
- fainting

This chapter has covered the development of your importance as a pharmacy technician, patients' expectations, tools needed to properly evaluate drugs, and a means to understand the importance of symptoms and their combinations. Most importantly, as a pharmacy technician you provide patients with an extraordinary service. Where pharmacists move on to new specialties, you must fill the gap. It will be your competence which inspires patients' confidence.

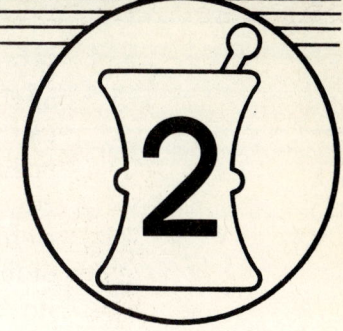

The Drug Order

The activities of the pharmacy technician begin after a patient has been seen by the physician, the physician has made a diagnosis requiring medication to remedy the ailment, and a prescription order is written communicating the physician's drug of choice, to be prepared by the pharmacy. If the illness is not severe enough to require hospitalization, the physician may order a medication which the patient fills at his or her local pharmacy. The nonhospitalized patient is regarded as ambulatory, as opposed to being hospitalized or an inpatient. Severe or complicated illnesses usually require a hospital stay, in which case the physician orders specific services and medications on a hospital form called the *Physician's Order*.

This chapter deals with prescriptions (often referred to as the *script*) written for ambulatory patients, as well as Physician's Orders. These are the two primary methods used to notify the hospital pharmacy or the retail pharmacy what specific medications are needed, the quantities requested, and the directions for their use. The information contained on the orders and scripts represents the result of the physician's diagnosis, which is based on his or her training, experience, and test results.

The term *physician* or *doctor* in this text refers to any practitioner legally permitted to prescribe drugs. He or she may be a medical doctor, osteopath, dentist, podiatrist, or veterinarian. For brevity, the terms will be used interchangeably.

Realizing the training and expertise that supports the diagnosis made by a physician, the pharmacy technician must carefully exercise his or her knowledge of drugs and dispensing, assuring that no misinterpretation occurs regarding the strength, the amount to be given, or the directions for use by each patient. Figures 2-1 and 2-2 illustrate examples of a blank script and a hospital Physician's Order. The composition of medication orders indicates that a specific battery of knowledge and skills are necessary in order to prepare and dispense the patient's medications properly. You will see that a basic understanding of mathematics, a knowledge of the Latin terms relevant to pharmacy, an ability to work with mathematical conversions, and a knowledge of what should be contained on pharmacy orders are needed to perform your role as a pharmacy technician appropriately.

Practicing pharmacy competently requires that you learn and use the "tools of the trade," and understand the abbreviations and terminology used frequently by medical and medical-support personnel. The patient's well-being is your primary concern. You must never leave any question unanswered by assumption.

NEVER DISPENSE GUESSWORK

Keep this phrase in mind, and make it part of your daily practice. Pharmacy should not be just "counting, pouring, licking, and sticking."

THE SCRIPT

The traditional prescription follows a definite pattern, which is intended to assure patient safety and legal compliance. Although the format has changed somewhat over the years, certain information is

```
1  PAT SMITH, M.D.
2  27 Oak Leaf Lane
   Baltimore, MD  12121
3  Phone: 322-7890       Name_____  4

                        Address_____
                                         Age_____  5

7      Rx
                                                   8
                                                   9
                                                   10

   [ ] Contents are labeled   May be refilled 0 1 2 3 4   11
       unless checked
                              Signed_____M.D.  12
6                             Date_____ 19__ DEA No.__ 13
```

Figure 2-1 The script.

PATIENT:
AGE:
SEX:
RACE:
CHART NO.

MEMORIAL HOSPITAL
BALTIMORE, MARYLAND
PHYSICIAN'S ORDER RECORD

BEAR DOWN ON HARD SURFACE WITH BALL POINT PEN

GENERIC EQUIVALENT IS AUTHORIZED UNLESS CHECKED IN THIS COLUMN

ALLERGY OR SENSITIVITY
TO
NONE KNOWN ☐ SIGNED:

DIAGNOSIS

COMPLETED OR DISCONTINUED

	DATE	TIME	ORDERS	PHYSICIAN'S SIG.		NAME	DATE	TIME

PHARMACY COPY

Figure 2-2 The Physician's Order.

necessary in order to prepare the medication properly. You may not expect to find the "Rx" superscription, but you certainly will need to know the drug prescribed, its strength, and the directions for using the drug.

Major Elements

Referring to the model prescription order in Figure 2-1, note the major elements contained on the ideal prescription:

1. prescriber's name and title (MD, DDS, DMD, DO, etc.)
2. prescriber's office address
3. prescriber's phone number
4. patient's name and address
5. patient's age
6. date on which the prescription was written
7. superscription (The Rx is Latin for "Take Thou.")
8. drug name, strength, and form (technically known as the *inscription* or body of the prescription)
9. quantity of the drug to be dispensed (known as the *subscription*)
10. clearly written and understandable directions (technically called the *signature*). *Note:* Although directions may be written in Latin abbreviations by the prescriber, directions to the patient must be spelled out in English. The directions should contain the amount of medication to be taken, the frequency, and the route of administration. The directions may also contain the reason for the medication (for example, for pain, for infection) if the prescriber so indicates.
11. refill instructions
12. prescriber's signature
13. prescriber's DEA number, which is required for prescriptions containing controlled drug substances. *Note:* DEA refers to the Drug Enforcement Administration, which is a federal agency within the Department of Justice. This arm of the law oversees controlled drug substances traffic. Controlled drugs, controlled substances, or controlled drug substances (CDS) refer to those drugs which possess a high potential for abuse (for example, diazepam, codeine, chloral hydrate).

Upon receipt of a properly written script (see Figure 2-3), you are able to prepare or "fill" the prescription without guesswork. In addition, a properly written script also enables you to dispense the medication to the patient in a timely manner. In reality, however, the ideal prescription rarely exists. You will find that it is necessary to examine the script closely, questioning the patient at times and perhaps phoning the doctor for clarification. There are a number of customary things to look for, and questions to ask:

The Script

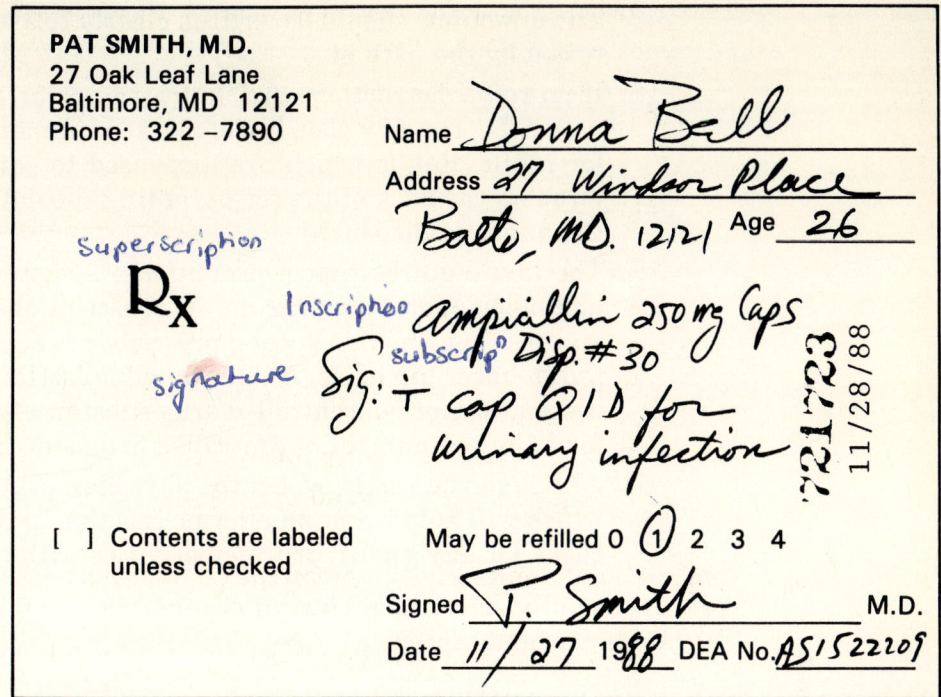

Figure 2-3

1. Is this a legitimate prescription blank with the practitioner's name, address, and phone number clearly written on the blank?
2. Is the full name of the patient written on the prescription? (Patient's initials should not be acceptable, inasmuch as this presents a potential for errors.)
3. Check the date the prescription was written. This is important because controlled substances should not be filled or refilled (if refills are indicated) more than six months after the script is issued to the patient.
4. The patient's address is a legal requirement for prescriptions containing a controlled drug substance. It is a good practice to complete the address on ALL prescriptions. Many potential errors may be avoided in those cases where family common names occur frequently, or specific names are customary for a particular region.
5. Does the drug, the strength, and the form requested by the practitioner appear on the script? Old drugs with new modifications or uses as well as new drugs are constantly entering the market. Make an effort to establish the drug's existence, and if necessary, contact the doctor if you are unclear regarding the medication.
6. Does the quantity seem adequate? For example, you may question the quantity if a practitioner prescribes an antibiotic for an extremely long period of time, or an antitubercular drug for a very short duration. Learn what the customary course of treatment is for the most common ailments.

7. The directions should be written clearly to avoid any misinterpretation by the patient.
8. If no refill instructions are indicated on the prescription, permit *no refills*. The law clearly defines requirements and time frames for refills. Refills which are dispensed to patients should be entered on the back of the script, noting the date, your initials, and the quantity dispensed.
9. The law requires that a practitioner's signature, DEA number, and office address appear on all prescriptions for controlled substances. You should expect a prescriber to sign prescriptions written in his or her office. A telephoned prescription does not require a signature for noncontrolled drug substances. This also holds true for a limited number of controlled drug substances.
10. Although you would expect the physician to prescribe medications which will not trigger an allergic reaction in the sensitive patient, check for any known drug sensitivities with the patient.

A carefully screened prescription order can avoid many unnecessary problems and confusion.

Problem Areas

Some areas tend to be more prone to error than others. The following discussion highlights some of these areas.

Last Name Only (Patient). A prescription will often be presented with only the last name of the patient. You must be sure that the prescription is being prepared for the person for whom it is intended. Therefore, it may be necessary to verify the prescription with the patient.

Use of an Initial Rather than a Complete First Name (Patient). This situation can be as harmful as the "last name only" circumstance unless a family profile is maintained by the pharmacy. Use of a letter initial can become a problem even on a family profile if more than one member of the family have first names beginning with the same initial. You should not assume who the patient is, but check with the family or doctor's office.

Address. The patient's address is especially important when a number of customers share a common name, when the prescription is to be billed, or when an insurance company is the payer. The address also serves as a check to assure that the person for whom the prescription was intended receives the medication.

Age. The age of the patient is important where dosages are crucial. Age is also important where dosage forms (liquids, capsules, tablets, ointments, suppositories, etc.) vary for a particular drug. It is not uncommon for a "rushed" practitioner to prescribe capsules or tablets for children who are too young to swallow solid dosage forms.

Date on Which the Prescription Was Written. Undated prescriptions present another problem. The consequence of having an undated prescription order is that the original condition for which the prescription was written may be different from some recently self-diagnosed condition for which the patient is now using the original, unfilled prescription. Some pharmacies may require a new prescription, or verbal confirmation from the doctor, in order to continue an old prescription order beyond six months.

Legibility. There is no doubt that legibility is the greatest offending factor in prescription error. In order to avoid dispensing guesswork, check with the pharmacist (since he or she is legally responsible for any errors committed by technicians), or with the prescribing practitioner. When questioning the prescription, ask the pharmacist or physician what the prescription reads, rather than asking if the illegible writing is a particular drug. Naming the drug or suggesting the directions (directions are also a cause for question) tends to bias the prescribing practitioner, taking away the total objectivity needed to decipher the illegibility.

Lack of a DEA Number. The Drug Enforcement Administration (DEA) issues a recorded registry number (DEA number) to eligible practitioners to be used when writing prescriptions for controlled drugs or narcotics. The DEA number is not required on prescriptions for drugs other than narcotics or controlled drugs. When you complete a controlled drug substance prescription, make it evident that the prescription contained a controlled substance by stamping or putting a red-colored "C" on the blank. All prescription forms for controlled substances must also contain the patient's full name and complete address, in addition to the DEA number of the doctor.

Clarity of Directions. Legibility has already been addressed. The clarity in this case refers to the intent of the directions. How does a practitioner want the patient to take the medication? The most abused direction is "Take as Directed" (often seen on the prescription order as ut. dict., u.d., ud, or as dir.). Although "Take as Directed" is not a satisfactory direction, it is not your position to interpret the doctor's intent, since this is between the patient and the doctor, based on the doctor's examination and diagnosis. If you see a blatant error that may be harmful, you can be sure that this was not the intent of the practitioner. Type the directions as you perceive them to be for the best use of the drug and the greatest benefit to the patient. However, when asked by the patient how to take the drug, or when left with a feeling that the patient is unsure of the directions, simply ask the patient how the doctor told him or her to take the medication. Should there continue to be any uncertainty, you may call the practitioner's office for clarification, or have the patient reaffirm the instructions with his or her doctor.

Another common direction which confuses many people involves taking the drug while awake (during waking hours) or around the clock (for example, "Take one capsule every four hours"). If there is any doubt regarding how the drug should be taken, first check the literature for specific details. If nothing can be concluded from the information provided, you may be required to make the decision. The literature may set a limit on the amount to be taken (for example, "Do not take more than eight capsules in a twenty-four hour period"). In the absence of limitations or clarity documented in the literature, a rule of thumb to follow is that antibiotics should be taken around the clock (at least during the initial phase of twenty-four to forty-eight hours), pain medications (analgesics) may be taken over a twenty-four hour period if the patient is awake and the pain is severe enough to require the medication. Other drugs, such as antihistamines, tranquilizers, antidepressants, anti-inflammatory drugs, and so on, should be limited to waking hours. This position may be taken when directions specify a number of times a day (for example, "Take one tablet three times a day").

Refill Instructions. If no mention is made of refills, it is safe to assume that no refills were intended. Should the patient insist that the practitioner said refills were allowed, you may agree with the patient (depending on the type of drug being ordered—be careful with controlled drug substances), and verify refill instructions with the doctor at a more convenient time.

The Prescription Label

Once you are satisfied with the contents of the prescription and are confident that the information provided enables you to fill the prescription without guesswork, you are ready to fill the order and prepare a label identifying the patient and instructing the patient how to take the medication. Ideally, the label should contain specific information, as illustrated in Figure 2-4. Referring to Figure 2-4, review the contents of the label:

1. a prescription serial number (referred to as the Rx number) and the date the prescription order is filled
2. the patient's full name
3. clearly typed instructions for taking the medication. *Note:* The first word of the directions should infer the route of administration. For example:
   internal/oral route—"Take"
   eye/ear/nose—"Instill" or "Place"
   topical lotion/ointment—"Apply"
   rectal/vaginal—"Insert"
4. the name of the drug (called labeling), unless specifically requested by the practitioner not to label
5. the pharmacist's initials and the initials of the pharmacy technician who prepared the drug for dispensing
6. the practitioner's name

The Physician's Order

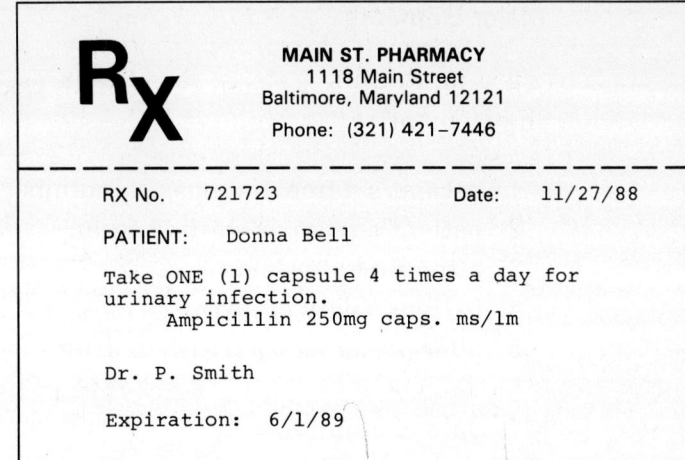

Figure 2-4 The prescription label.

```
FINISH ALL THIS MEDICATION
UNLESS OTHERWISE DIRECTED
BY PRESCRIBER
```

```
REFILL ONE TIME
```

```
TAKE ON AN EMPTY STOMACH
ONE HOUR BEFORE MEALS OR
TWO HOURS AFTER MEALS
```

Figure 2-5 Strip labels.

7. the drug's expiration date
8. Additional labels, called "strip" labels (for example, TAKE WITH FOOD OR MILK, DO NOT TAKE WITH ALCOHOL, TAKE ON AN EMPTY STOMACH), may be applied to the bottle containing the medication, informing the patient of a particular way to take the drug which would assure the medication's optimal effect. See Figure 2-5 for additional examples.
9. the number of refills, if any, or *no refills*, if none

THE PHYSICIAN'S ORDER

The basic principles and care undertaken to examine the ambulatory patient's prescription order also apply to the Physician's Order (illustrated in Figure 2-2) for the hospitalized patient, even though all the script elements discussed do not appear on the Physician's Order. Screening the drug, the strength, the directions for use, and the patient for whom the medication is intended may be more important in the hospital setting, inasmuch as the variety of drugs and the forms for different routes of administration are more numerous and potentially more dangerous than those found in the local retail pharmacy.

Major Elements

An appropriately written Physician's Order should contain the following elements:

1. patient's name and hospital number
2. patient's room or ward location
3. attending physician
4. patient's date of birth
5. allergies or sensitivities to drugs, foods, etc.
6. diagnosis
7. date of admission
8. patient's condition
9. services to be performed (that is, tests, activities, diet, etc.)
10. medications
11. strength of each medication
12. dosage form (tablet, liquid, suppository, injectable, etc.) Dosage form is specified in order to avoid any question regarding the form to be given. For example, nurses prefer to administer drugs in liquid form to patients who have nasogastric tubes, and suppositories or injection are generally used in vomiting patients. Most drugs come prepared in more than one dosage form. Although dosage form is not often written, you can interpret the most appropriate form to use by looking for keynotes such as NGT (nasogastric tube) or age.
13. directions for the use or frequency of administration for each medication
14. nurse's or physician's signature and time of entry on the Physician's Order

You should be completely certain of what is wanted, for whom it is ordered, and how it is to be given. Remember, NEVER DISPENSE GUESSWORK.

Most hospitals have a listing of drugs, referred to as a *drug formulary*. The drugs included in the formulary are those medicinal agents which have been reviewed by the hospital's Pharmacy Therapeutics Committee (PT Committee), and have been recommended for inventory based on their therapeutic benefits and economy. Occasionally, only one specific dosage form or strength of a drug will be included in the formulary. Although hospital formularies exist to control costs by limiting the drug inventory, nonformulary drugs may usually be ordered for a particular patient if requested by the prescriber.

Hospital pharmacies usually adopt an automatic stop order policy. The automatic stop order (ASO) may vary for the different categories of drugs for each hospital. For instance, standing orders (those medications ordered by the physician which can be presumed to be continued as long as the patient is in the hospital) may specify an automatic stop for narcotics after seventy-two hours. Therefore, the pharmacy will acknowledge and dispense no more than seventy-two hours worth of the drug. A physician would be required to reorder the narcotic after this time. In many hospitals, standing orders are automatically stopped when the patient undergoes surgery or is transferred to another part of the hospital.

The PRN (*Pro Re Nata*, Latin for "as needed") category of drugs refers to the medications which are not used routinely, but only when they are needed. Some examples of this category are nonnarcotic pain medications (for example, acetaminophen, propoxyphene), sleeping agents (for example, flurazepam, temazepam), and laxatives. It is your task to learn what the stop order policies are for the specific hospital where you are employed.

COMMON PHARMACEUTICAL NOTATIONS

Hospital staffs generally adopt commonly used abbreviations. Occasionally, however, practitioners may develop their own form of shorthand which is limited to use only in those hospitals in which they are working. Tables 2-1 through 2-4 provide the pharmacy and drug abbreviations commonly used in hospitals, as well as generally accepted medical abbreviations. Concerning those special abbreviations found only within a specific hospital, question their meaning when you have the slightest doubt. Once you determine their meaning, note it in a personal resource file to be used as a reference source when needed.

TABLE 2-1

Common Abbreviations Used in Medical Orders

Abbreviation	Meaning
$\overline{aa}$, aa	of each
a.c.	before meals
ad	to, up to
a.d.	right ear
ad lib.	at pleasure, as desired
a.l.	left ear
A.M.	morning
aq.	water
aq. dest.	distilled water
a.s.	left ear
a.u.	each ear
b.i.d., bd	twice a day
b.m.	bowel movement
b.p.	blood pressure
C	one hundred
$\overline{c}$, c	with
caps.	capsules
comp.	compound
d.	day
dil.	dilute
disp.	dispense
div.	divide
d.t.d.	give of such a dose
el., elix.	elixir
et	and
f., ft.	make, let be made

TABLE 2-1 (*Continued*)

Abbreviation	Meaning
Gm., g.	gram
gr.	grain
gtt., gtts.	a drop, drops
h.	hour
h.s., hor. som.	at bedtime
IM	intramuscular
IV	intravenously
liq.	liquid, solution
M.	mix
m. dict.	as directed
mixt., mist.	a mixture
no.	number
noc., N, n	night
non. rep.	do not repeat, no refills
O, Oct.	a pint
o.d.	right eye
o.l.	left eye
o.s.	left eye
o.u.	each eye or both eyes
p.c., post. cib.	after meals
P.M.	evening
p.o.	by mouth, orally
p.r.	rectally
p.r.n.	as needed
pulv.	a powder
q	every
qAM	every morning
qd	every day
qh	every hour
q.i.d.	four times a day
q.o.d.	every other day
qPM	every evening
q.s., qs ad	a sufficient quantity, up to
q.v.	as much as you wish
Rx	take, take thou, a recipe, prescription
rep.	let it be repeated
s̄, s	without
s.a.	according to the art (secundum artem)
sat.	saturated
Sig.	label, let it be printed (signa)
sol.	solution
s.q., SQ	subcutaneous
s̄s, ss	one-half
s.o.s.	if there is a need
stat	at once, immediately
subq	subcutaneously
supp.	suppository
syr.	syrup
tab.	tablet
t.i.d.	three times a day
tr., tinct.	tincture
trit.	triturate
ung.	ointment
ut. dict., u.d., ud	as directed
w.a.	while awake
X	ten

Common Pharmaceutical Notations

TABLE 2-2

Common Symbols Used in Medical Orders

Symbol	Meaning
℥	teaspoonful
℥	2 tablespoonsful, 1 fluid ounce, 30 milliliters
℥ss	1 tablespoonful, 15 milliliters
Ⓛ	left
Ⓡ	right
ϕ	none
Δ	change
>	greater than
<	less than
↑	increase
↓	decrease
'	minutes
"	seconds
°	hours
1°	primary
2°	secondary

TABLE 2-3

Common Drug Abbreviations

Abbreviation	Trade Name	Generic Name	Use
$AgNO_3$	none	silver nitrate	anti-infective
APAP	Tylenol	acetaminophen	analgesic
ASA	Ecotrin	aspirin	analgesic
bicarb	none	bicarbonate (sodium)	antacid/electrolyte
B-1	Betalin S	thiamine	vitamin
B-6	Hexa-Betalin	pyridoxine	vitamin
B-12	Rubramin PC	cyanocobalamin	vitamin
Ca	Ca-Plus	calcium	nutritional supplement
CaCl	none	calcium chloride	electrolyte
$CaCO_3$	Os-Cal	calcium carbonate	nutritional supplement
CT	Chlor-Trimeton	chlorpheniramine	antihistamine
DC	Darvon Compound	propoxyphene, aspirin, caffeine	analgesic
DES	Stilphostrol	diethylstilbesterol	hormone
DHE	D.H.E. 45	dihydroergotamine	vasoconstrictor
dig, digox	Lanoxin	digoxin	cardiac drug
DPH	Benadryl	diphenhydramine	antihistamine
	Dilantin	diphenylhydantoin (generic name changed to phenytoin)	anticonvulsant
DPT	Triogen	diphtheria, pertussis, and tetanus	vaccine
DSS	Colace	dioctyl sodium sulfosuccinate	laxative
D_5S	none	5% dextrose in saline	intravenous fluid
D_5W	none	5% dextrose in water	intravenous fluid
epi	Adrenalin	epinephrine	bronchodilator/heart stimulant
ETH	none	elixir terpin hydrate	expectorant
ETH c. Cod	none	elixir terpin hydrate with codeine	expectorant/cough suppressant
ETOH	none	ethanol/ethyl alcohol	skin disinfectant
F.A.	Folvite	folic acid	vitamin
$FeSO_4$	Feosol	ferrous sulfate	iron supplement
gent	Garamycin	gentamicin	antibiotic

TABLE 2-3 (Continued)

Abbreviation	Trade Name	Generic Name	Use
GG	Robitussin	glyceryl guaiacolate, guaifenesin	expectorant
HC	Cortef	hydrocortisone	steroid
HCTZ	Oretic	hydrochlorothiazide	diuretic
H_2O	none	water	fluid
H_2O_2	none	hydrogen peroxide	antiseptic
INH	INH	Isoniazid	antitubercular
KCl	Kay Ciel	potassium chloride	electrolyte
KI	SSKI	potassium iodide	expectorant
KISS	SSKI	saturated solution of potassium iodide	expectorant
KPO_4	Neutra-Phos	potassium phosphate	electrolyte
LCD	Zetar	coal tar solution	antipruritic
L-Dopa	Larodopa	levodopa	anti-Parkinson
$LiCO_3$	Eskalith	lithium carbonate	psychotherapeutic drug
LR	none	lactated ringers solution	intravenous fluid
mag. cit.	none	magnesium citrate	laxative
mgO	none	magnesium oxide	antacid/laxative
$mgSO_4$	none	magnesium sulfate	anticonvulsant
m.o.	Kondremul	mineral oil	laxative
MOM	none	milk of magnesia	antacid/laxative
MS	none	morphine sulfate	analgesic
MVI	many	multiple vitamins	vitamins
NaCl	none	sodium chloride	electrolyte
$NaHCO_3$, NaBicarb.	none	sodium bicarbonate	antacid/electrolyte
$NaPO_4$	K-Phos	sodium phosphate	electrolyte
NS, NSS	none	normal saline solution	intravenous fluid
PABA	Pabanol	para-aminobenzoic acid	sunscreen
PBZ	Pyribenzamine	tripelennamine	antihistamine
Pb, phenobarb	SK-Phenobarbital	phenobarbital	sedative
PCN	none	penicillin	antibiotic
PCN G	Pfizerpen	penicillin G	antibiotic
PCN VK	Veetids	penicillin VK	antibiotic
pit	Pitocin	oxytocin	hormone
PPD	Aplisol	purified protein derivative	tuberculin test
PTU	none	propylthiouracil	antithyroid
PZI	none	protamine zinc insulin	blood glucose regulator
RL	none	ringer's lactate	intravenous fluid
sal acid	Keralyt	salicylic acid	keratolytic
SSKI	SSKI	saturated solution of potassium iodide	expectorant
TCN	Sumycin	tetracycline	antibiotic
TNG	Nitrostat	nitroglycerin	antianginal
tobra	Nebcin	tobramycin	antibiotic
TSH	Thytropar	thyroid stimulating hormone	hormone
Vit. C	Cevi-Bid	ascorbic acid	vitamin
Vit. K	Synkavite Mephyton	menadiol phytonadione	vitamin
ZnO	none	zinc oxide	protectant
$ZnSO_4$	Zinc-220	zinc sulfate	nutritional supplement

Common Pharmaceutical Notations

TABLE 2-4

Common Hospital Abbreviations

Abbreviation	Meaning
ABD	abdomen
abd prep	abdominal preparation
ABG	arterial blood gases
AC lab	anticoagulation laboratory
ACT	activity
ADA	American Dietetic Association
AK	above knee
alk phos	alkaline phosphatase
all	allergy
AMA	against medical advice
amp	ampule
antibio	antibiotics
AP chest	anteroposterior chest X-ray
APhA	American Pharmaceutical Association
ASAP	as soon as possible
ASCVD	arteriosclerotic cardiovascular disease
ASHD	arteriosclerotic heart disease
ASHP	American Society of Hospital Pharmacists
ASO	automatic stop order
BE	barium enema
bili	bilirubin
BK	below knee
BM	bowel movement
BMR	basal metabolic rate
BP	blood pressure
BRP	bathroom privileges
BSA	body surface area
BSS	buffered saline solution
BUN	blood urea nitrogen
C	gallon or the Roman numeral for 100
C&S	culture and sensitivity
C.A.	continuous action
CA	cancer
cap	capsule
cath	catheter
CBC	complete blood count
CBC c. diff	complete blood count with differentials
cc	cubic centimeter
CCU	coronary care unit
CDS	controlled drug substance
Chest AP	see AP chest
CHF	congestive heart failure
CICU	coronary intensive care unit
CLD, CL diet	clear liquid diet
cond	condition
cont	continuous
COPD	chronic obstructive pulmonary disease
C section	Cesarean section
CSF	cerebral spinal fluid
CVA	cerebrovascular accident
CXR	chest X-ray
cysto	cystoscopy
D.A.	delayed action
DC, D/C	discontinue or discharge
DEA	Drug Enforcement Administration
decub	decubitus
dig	digoxin

TABLE 2-4 (Continued)

Abbreviation	Meaning
dig level	digoxin blood level
DR	delivery room
DS	double strength
DSD	dry sterile dressing
Dx	diagnosis
E.C.	enteric coated
ECG or EKG	electrocardiogram
EEG	electroencephalogram
ER	emergency room
FBS	fasting blood sugar
FDA	Food and Drug Administration
Fe	iron
FiO$_2$	frequency of inspired air
FS	floor stock
FTT	failure to thrive
FUO	fever of unknown origin
Fx	fracture
F(x)	function
GFR	glomerular filtration rate
GI	gastrointestinal
gluc	glucose
Gm., gm., G.	gram
gr.	grain
gtt.	drop(s)
GU	genitourinary
GYN	gynecology
H.A. or HA	headache
HCl	hydrochloride
Hct	hematocrit
HCVD	hypertensive cardiovascular disease
HEENT	head, eye, ear, nose, throat
Hep Lock, H.L.	heparin lock
Hg	mercury
Hgb	hemoglobin
H.O.	house officer
H.P.	high potency
HR	heart rate or hyperalimentation rate
H.T.	hypodermic tablet
HTFN	hold till further notice
Hx	history
Hyperal, HAL	hyperalimentation
I&O	intake and output
ICN	intensive care nursery
ICU	intensive care unit
I.M.	intramuscular
IP	inpatient
IPPB	intermitten positive pressure breathing
IU	international unit
IUD	intrauterine device
IUP	intrauterine pregnancy
I.V.	intravenous
IVF	intravenous fluids
IVP	intravenous pyelogram
IVR	intravenous rate
JCAH	Joint Commission on Accreditation of Hospitals

TABLE 2-4 (Continued)

Abbreviation	Meaning
K⁺ level	potassium level
KO	keep open
KVO	keep vein open
L	liter
L.A.	long acting
LAS	label as such
lat	lateral
LDH	lactodehydrogenase
L.E.	lupus erythematosus
LFT	liver function test
LOA	leave of absence
LOC	laxative of choice
LPN	licensed practical nurse
lytes	electrolytes
M&M enema	milk and molasses enema
Mcg., mcg.	microgram
meds	medications
mEq.	milliequivalent
Mg., mg.	milligram
MI	myocardial infarction
MIC	minimum inhibitory concentration
ml.	milliliter
MLD	minimum lethal dose
mm.	millimeter
MN	midnight
N, NL	normal
Na⁺ level	sodium level
narc	narcotic
N.B.	note well, take notice
NBN	newborn nursery
NC	nasal cannula
NDC	National Drug Code
NGT, NG tube	nasogastric tube
NH	nursing home
NICU	newborn intensive care unit
NKA	no known allergies
NKDA	no known drug allergy
NKMA	no known medication allergy
NPO	nothing by mouth
NS	normal saline
nst	not sent
n/v	nausea and vomiting
O	pint
OB	obstetrics
OD	overdose
OJ	orange juice
oint.	ointment
OP	outpatient
opth.	ophthalmic
OOB	out of bed
OR	operating room
P	per, after
P.A.	prolonged action
PA	posteroanterior X-ray, physician's assistant
PBI	protein-bound iodine
PDR	Physician's Desk Reference
Peds	pediatrics

TABLE 2-4 (Continued)

Abbreviation	Meaning
PFT	pulmonary function test
PKU	phenylketonuria
p.o.	by mouth (occasionally "phone order")
Port	portable
post-op	after surgery
PP	post prandial, post partum
ppm	parts per million
pr	per rectum
PRBC	packed red blood cells
pre-op	before surgery
pt.	patient
PT	physical therapy, prothrombin time (test for coumadin)
PTT	prothrombin time (test for heparin)
PVB	premature ventricular beat
PVC	premature ventricular contraction
R&M	routine and microscopy
R.A.	released action
RBC	red blood cell
Reg	regular
R.N.	registered nurse
ROM	range of motion
R/O	rule out
RR	recovery room
RTC	return to clinic
RTS	return to stock
S.A.	sustained action or slow-acting
S.C.	sugar coated
sc	subcutaneous
SGOT	serum glutamic oxaloacetic transaminase
SGPT	serum glutamic pyruvic transaminase
s.l.	sublingual
SMA	serial multiple analysis
SOB	shortness of breath
sono	sonogram
S/P	status post, state of a condition
sp. gr.	specific gravity
S.R.	sustained release, slow release
STAT	immediately
supp	suppository
SQ, sq	subcutaneous
T, temp	temperature
T>	temperature greater than
tach	tachycardia
T&A	tonsillectomy and adenoidectomy
TXC	type and crossmatch
TB	tuberculosis
tbsp	tablespoonful
T.D.	timed disintegrating
tele	telemetry
TIA	transient ischemic attack
TLC	tender loving care
TO	transfer orders
TPR	temperature, pulse, respiration
T.R.	timed release
trans	transfer
TRH	thyrotropin releasing hormone
TSH	thyroid stimulating hormone
tsp	teaspoonful

Common Pharmaceutical Notations

TABLE 2-4 (Continued)

Abbreviation	Meaning
T.T.	tablet triturate
TUR	transurethral resection
TV	total volume
TX	treatment
u	unit
U/A, UA	urinalysis
UGI	upper gastrointestinal series
URI	upper respiratory infection
USP	United States Pharmacopeia
UTI	urinary tract infection
VDRL	venereal disease research laboratory
VO	verbal order
VS	vital signs
w.a.	while awake
WBC	white blood cells

Medical Terminology

WORD DEVELOPMENT: USAGE AND COMPONENTS

Language is the foundation of communication. Jargon is language that is special to a geographical area, social class, age group, or occupation.

As a pharmacy technician, you should be familiar with where and how a drug works. In order to properly understand the workings of any drug, you must have a basic medical/pharmaceutical vocabulary. You are not expected to know the meaning of every medical term used in anatomy, physiology, or disease condition. Likewise, it is impossible to know every pharmacy term used to express drug activities or sites of action.

Learning some basic principles behind the process of forming medical terms from components will enable you to dissect any word, understand it, and use it appropriately. This chapter addresses word components, their meanings, and word formation.

In medicine, most words follow a general equation for their development:

$$\text{Prefix} + \text{Root} + \text{Suffix} = \text{Word}$$

(*Note:* You may not always find these three parts in every medical word. In most cases, however, you should find a root and suffix.) The parts of the word are called its components. The prefix usually tells where and how or what. The prefix *sub-*, for example, notes "below" or "less than," as in the word *subcutaneous*, meaning "beneath the skin." *Tachy-* in *tachycardia* is telling you how the heart is beating or contracting. Tachycardia denotes an increase or acceleration (*tachy* meaning "rapid or swift") in the heart rate.

The root portion of a medical term tells you what system is being affected. Refer to our previous examples—subcutaneous and tachycardia. The root portion, *cut* in subcutaneous refers to skin which is part of the integumentary system (this anatomical system includes skin, hair, nails, sweat glands, and sebaceous glands). *cardi* in tachycardia is a cardiovascular system root component referring to the heart.

Suffixes may be categorized as diagnostic (for example, *-itis*, indicating a reddening or inflammation), symptomatic (for example, *-algia*, expressing a pain symptom), or operative (for example, *-ectomy*, denoting an excision or "cutting out"). There are many suffixes which may be interpreted differently and cross over these categories. You may question whether a suffix really belongs in a selected category. For the purposes of this text we merely want to grasp some basic principles involved in word formation. This chapter will enable you to develop an ability to break down most medical and pharmacy terms successfully and understand their appropriate meanings. Experience and exposure to more words through your readings will also help you develop your own subcategories which you will use to define many words.

You will avoid error and confusion by interpreting medical and pharmaceutical terms from right to left. For example, the word *antibiotic* has a definite prefix, root, and suffix. Reading from right to left, note the following:

suffix: (*t*)*ic*—*t* = one of a number of letters used to connect the components of medical terms. *ic* means "pertaining to."
root: *bio*—means "life"
prefix: *anti*—means "against"

An anitibiotic, literally defined, expresses something that is against life or interferes with life. In fact, an antibiotic is an agent which is used to destroy or interfere with the development of harmful organisms (often called pathogenic bacteria).

Let's look at a more complex medical term which, dissected from left to right, results in a wrong meaning: *osteomalacia*.

Osteomalacia, broken down into its components from left to right, looks like this:

oste—oma—lacia

oste—denotes "bone"
oma—refers to tumors
lacia—this component becomes meaningless

The resulting definition for this word, based on a left-to-right interpretation, erroneously leads you to believe this word refers to a bone tumor.

Correctly broken down from right to left, however, the word becomes:

oste—o—malacia

malacia—"softening of a part"
o—a component-combining letter
oste—denoting "bone"

You now have the true definition of *osteomalacia*—"bone softening."

The components in Figure 3-1 and in Tables 3-1 through 3-12 will provide a good foundation upon which to build a solid vocabulary. Always check with any of a number of medical dictionaries for less often used words or components and enter them in your personal reference file.

Sounds of Letter Combinations

Letter Combination	Sound
ch	k
cn	n
gn	n
ph	f
pn	n
ps	s
rh	r

Examples:

chelation sounds like "kelation"
cnemis sounds like "nemis"
gnathion sounds like "nathion"
pharmacy sounds like "farmacy"
pneumonia sounds like "neumonia"
psychogenic sounds like "syckogenic"
rhinitis sounds like "rynitis"

Pluralization

Singular	Plural
-a	-ae
-ex	-ces
-is	-es
-on	-a
-um	-a
-us	-i
-itis	-itides

Figure 3-1 Letter combination sounds and pluralization.

Word Development: Usage and Components

TABLE 3-1

Common Prefixes in Medical Terminology

Prefix	Meaning	Example
a-, an-	lacking	anemia
ab-	away from	abnormal
ad-	above, on top of	adrenal
ambi-	denoting two	ambidexterous
amphi-	around	amphicrania
ana-	up, back again	anabiosis
ante-	just before	antepartum
anti-	oppose, against	antibiotic
apo-	away, separation	apocrine
bi-	two	bilateral
brady-	slow	bradycardia
cata-	down, downward, against	catabolism
contra-	against, opposite	contraceptive
de-	preventing, away from	desensitize
di-	referring to two	dichromatopsia
dia-	through	diaphoresis
dis-	apart, separation	dislocation
dys-	difficult	dyspnea
e-, ec-, ex-, es-	away from, beyond	exophthalmus
ecto-	outside, outer part	ectoretina
extra-	outside, beyond	extrarenal
erythro-	redness	erythrocyte
glyco-	sweetness	glycosuria
hemi-	half	hemigastrectomy
hyper-	excess	hypercalcemia
hypo-	deficiency	hypocalcemia
idio-	individual, distinct	idiopathic
infra-	below	infraorbital
intra-	within	intramuscular
juxta-	of close proximity	juxtacortical
lepto-	thin, narrow, mild, weakness	leptopellic
macro-	large	macroblepharia
meg-, magal-	huge, excessively large	megacolon
mesa-, meso-	middle	mesoderm
meta-	change, transformation	metabolism
micro-	very small	microgastria
olig-	very little	oliguria
omni-	all	omnivorous
pachy-	thickening	pachyostosis
para-	near	paracentesis
per-	puncture, through	percutaneous
peri-	around, enclosed	pericarditis
phaco-	denoting eye lens	phacohymenitis
poly-	excessive	polyuria
post-	after, behind	postclavicular
pre-	before, in front of	prechordal
pro-	before, in front of	prochondral
pseudo-	false	pseudoangina

TABLE 3-1 (*Continued*)

Prefix	Meaning	Example
py-, pyo-	denoting pus	pyorrhea
pyr-, pyreto	fever, heat	pyrogenic
re-	return, back, again	recalcification
retro-	backward	retroflexion
semi-	half	semipermeable
sclero-	hardening, stiffening	scleroderma
skeleto-	denoting the skeleton	skeletization
steno-	constriction, narrowing, shortening	stenocoriasis
sub-	less than, beneath	subcutaneous
super-	above	superalimentation
supra-	above	supranasal
sym-	with, along, beside	symbiosis
syn-	joined together	synanastomosis
tachy-	accelerated	tachycardia
trans-	across, in the process of change	transurethral
tri-	denoting three	triceps
ultra-	beyond, excess	ultraligation
un-	not, reversal	unconsciousness

TABLE 3-2

Common Roots in Terminology of the Cardiovascular System

Root	Meaning	Example
angi-	vessel, vein, artery	angioplasty
cardio-	heart	cardiomegaly
cardium-	heart	pericardium
cor-	heart	percordial
corona-	heart vessels	coronary
-cyte	cell	hematocyte
-emia	blood	hyperemia
hem-, heme-, hemato-	blood	hemapoiesis
lien-	spleen	lienocele
lymphaden-	lymph nodes	lymphadenitis
lymphangi-	lymph vessels	lymphangitis
phlebo-	denoting veins	phlebogenous
splen-	spleen	splenectasis
vas-, vaso-	vessel	vasoconstrictor
veni-, veno-	vein	venipuncture

Word Development: Usage and Components

TABLE 3-3

Common Roots in Terminology of the Digestive System

Root	Meaning	Example
arch-	anus	architis
bucca-	cheek	buccoversion
celi-	abdomen	celioma
cheil-	lip	cheilotomy
cholangi-	bile duct	cholangiectasis
cholecyst-	gallbladder	cholecystectomy
choledoch-	bile duct	choledocholithiasis
col-	large intestine	coloptosis
copro-	feces	coprolith
dento-	refers to teeth	dentoid
entero-	small intestine	enteritis
hepato-	liver	hepatitis
gastro-	stomach	gastritis
gingivo-	gums	gingivitis
gloss-	tongue	glossitis
gnatho-	jaw	gnathodynia
labi-	lip	labiomycosis
lapar-	abdominal wall	laparotomy
odont-	tooth	odontalgia
oro-, os-	mouth, opening	osculum
procto-	rectum	proctoscopy
ptyalo-	saliva	ptyalorrhea
recto-	denoting the rectum	rectoclysis
sial-	saliva	sialogogue
staphyl-	palate	staphyloptosis
stoma-, stomato-	opening, mouth	stomatalgia
ulo-	gums	uloglossitis
urano-	palate	uranoplasty

TABLE 3-4

Common Roots in Terminology of the Genito-urinary System

Root	Meaning	Example
colp-	vagina	colporrhagia
cyst-	bladder	cystoscopy
episio-	referring to the vulva	episiotomy
funicul-	small cord	funiculopexy
hyster-	uterus	hysterectomy
metro-	uterus	metrophlebitis
nephr-	kidney	nephrectomy
oophor-	ovary	oophorectomy
orchid-	testicles	orchidopexy
oscheo-	scrotum	oscheocele
pubio-, pubo-	pubic region	pubiotomy
pyel-	part of the kidney	pyelitis
ren-	kidney	renal
salping-	fallopian tubes	salpingostomy
spermo-, spermato-	denotes sperm	spermatocele
trachel-	cervix	trachelectomy
ur-, uro-, urono-	refers to urine and the urinary tract	uroclepsia
vesico-	refers to the urinary bladder	vesicotomy

TABLE 3-5

Common Roots in Terminology of the Integumentary System

Root	Meaning	Example
cut-	skin	subcutaneous
derma-, dermato-	skin	dermatitis
follic-	secretory sac	folliculoma
histo-	tissue	histoclastic
lipo-	refers to fat tissue	lipoblastoma
mamm-	breast	mammectomy
mast-	breast	mastodynia
onych-	nail	paronychia
pil-, pilo-	hair	pilonidal
sarco-	denotes flesh	sarcoadenoma
thel-	nipple	theleplasty
trich-, tricho-	hair	trichoglossia

TABLE 3-6

Common Roots in Terminology of the Musculo-skeletal system

Root	Meaning	Example
arthr-	joint	arthritis
cheiro-, chiro-	refers to the hand	cheirospasm
chondro-	cartilage	chondrodynia
cranio-	skull	craniopathy
facio-	refers to the face	facioplegia
leiomyo-	smooth muscle	leiomyoma
myelo-	marrow	osteomyelitis
myo-	skeletal muscle	myomalacia
os-	bone	osseous
osteo-	bone	osteoporosis
pod-	refers to the foot	pododynia
rhabdomyo-	striated muscle	rhabdomyanectomy
tendo-, teno-	tendons	tendinoplasty

TABLE 3-7

Common Roots in Terminology of the Nervous System

Root	Meaning	Example
cephal-	the head	cephalgia
cere-	brain	cerebrosclerosis
encephal-	within the head	encephalitis
meningo-	denotes membranes covering the brain and spinal cord	meningitis
ment-	mind	dementia
myel-	spinal cord	myelitis
neuro-	nerve	neuralgia
phren-	mind	phrenastenia
psych-	mind	psychosis
rach-	spinal column	rachialgia
spondyl-	vertebrae	spondylopathy

Word Development: Usage and Components

TABLE 3-8

Common Roots in Terminology of the Respiratory System

Root	Meaning	Example
broncho-	windpipe	bronchospasm
laryng-	voice box	laryngectomy
naso-	refers to the nose	nasosinusitis
-osmia	smell	hyperosmia
-pnea	act of breathing	dyspnea
pneumo-	lungs	pneumocentesis
pulmo-	lungs	pulmonitis
rhin-	nose	rhinitis
thoraco-	refers to the chest	thoracobronchotomy
trache-, tracheo-	air tube to lungs	tracheaectasis
trachelo-	denotes neck	trachelodynia

TABLE 3-9

Common Roots in Terminology of the Sense Organs

Root	Meaning	Example
auri-	ear	auripuncture
audit-	hearing	auditory
bleph-, blephar-	eyelid	blepharitis
dacryo-	tears	dacryagogue
dacryaden-	tear gland	dacryadenitis
dacryocyst-	tear sac	dacryocystocele
irid-	iris	iridectomy
derat-	cornea	keratitis
myring-	eardrum	myringotomy
oculo-	denoting the eye	oculomotor
ophthalm-	eye	ophthalmology
-opia	vision, sight	diplopia
optico-, opto-	relating to the eye or vision	opticopupillary
ot-	ear	otitis
palpebr-	eyelid	palpebral
phaco-	eye lens	phacoma

TABLE 3-10

Diagnostic Suffixes

Suffix	Meaning	Example
-cele	swelling, growing out	hydrocele
-ectasis	swelling, dilation	cardiectasis
-gram	tracing	electrocardiogram
-graph	record	encephalograph
-iasis	state or condition of, pathologic state	mydriasis
-itis	inflammation, reddening	gastritis
-malacia	softening	osteomalacia
-mania	irrational, madness	megalomania
-oid	denoting resemblance	carcinoid
-oma	denoting a tumor	dermatoma
-osis	denoting a deteriorating condition	osteomiosis
-pathy	a condition	dermatopathy
-phobia	fear	photophobia
-ptosis (pt = "t")	dropping, downward displacement	blepharoptosis
-rrhage, -rrhagia, -rrhagic	bursting forth	hemorrhage
-rrhea	flow	dysmenorrhea
-rrhexis	broken, burst	cardiorrhexis
-sthen, -sthenia	weakness	myasthenia

TABLE 3-11

Operative Suffixes

Suffix	Meaning	Example
-centesis	puncture	thoracentesis
-desis	binding	arthrodesis
-ectomy	excision, cutting out	gastrectomy
-oscopy	looking into	gastroscopy
-ostomy	making an opening	colostomy
-otomy	incision	gastrotomy
-pexy	fixing an organ in place	gastropexy
-plasty	shaping or forming	rhinoplasty
-rrhaphy	suture	gastrorrhaphy

TABLE 3-12

Symptomatic Suffixes

Suffix	Meaning	Example
-aemia, -emia	denoting blood	uremia
-algia	pain	myalgia
-dynia	pain	gastrodynia
-esthesia	denotes sensation	paresthesia
-genia	origin, production	myogenic
-osis	excessive	leukocytosis
-penia	lack	leukocytopenia
-trophy	denotes growth	hypertrophy

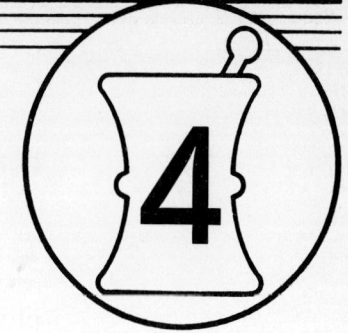

Basics of Human Functioning

AN OVERVIEW OF HUMAN ANATOMY AND PHYSIOLOGY

You may have heard stories of an individual living in a location highlighted by some outstanding landmark, such as the Empire State Building or the Golden Gate Bridge, who never avails himself or herself of the opportunity to see the famous structure which attracts so many. The same situation is true of our own bodies. Very few of us are familiar with our own body structure (anatomy) and the function of our systems (physiology). As a pharmacy technician, you must be familiar with this battery of knowledge about human anatomy and physiology, in order to appreciate where and how a drug works on a specifc region of the body. Familiarity with anatomy and function will help you to communicate and answer many questions patients ask. In addition, this information will help you achieve and maintain a professional position, credibility, and a working relationship with other members of the health care team, such as nurses, respiratory therapists, medical technicians, and so on.

A text of this dimension is intended to highlight the areas of anatomy and physiology which are useful to you as a pharmacy technician in your daily application to drug activities. If your interest and curiosity warrant further exploration of this area, many excellent texts are available.

By textbook definition, human anatomy is comprised of ten systems. Each system is composed of special parts or components. The role each system plays in maintaining functions and processes is referred to as *physiology*. When an abnormality occurs within a system or systems, the resulting condition is a disease state or disorder.

Cells: The Building Blocks

The primary structural building block of any anatomical system is the cell. Therefore, we will begin by briefly discussing the structure and physiology of the cell.

The branch of anatomy which deals with the study of cell structure and function is known as *cytology* (*cyt* = cell, *logy* = study of). Cells are the smallest units of living matter. They vary in size from those which can be seen only with the aid of an electron microscope, to those which can be seen with the naked eye. In addition to the variety of sizes, their shapes also differ.

All cells contain protein, carbohydrate, fat, nucleic acid (DNA and RNA), and other materials. Each cell is surrounded by a membrane called the *cell membrane*. This membrane assures that the cell remains intact. The cell membrane is made of a lipid (fat) layer surrounded by a protein layer. This composition of the cell membrane allows only certain substances to pass into the cell. This process of selective passage through the cell membrane is referred to as the *permeability* of a cell.

Inside the cell there are two major parts. The *nucleus* is the component responsible for cell activities and is considered the control center. The second major part is the living substance which surrounds the nucleus and is contained by the cell membrane. This material is known as *cytoplasm*. There are other structures in the cell, each having specialized functions in the cell's activities.

Groups of like cells form tissues, which form the organs. Therefore, all muscle cells are specific, all heart cells are specific, and so on. Reactions which are due to disease or drugs occur at the cell level. A drug being used to treat an abnormally functioning heart, for instance, passes through the heart cell membrane in order to create a response in the heart.

These masses of like cells form any of five basic tissues: epithelial (for example, skin), connective (for example, cartilage, bone), muscle, nerve, and blood. Tissues combine in specific arrangements to form organs (for example, heart, stomach, liver, brain). Finally, a group of organs join in a specialized manner, called a *system*, to perform a major function in the body.

Through physiologic processes, each system performs a role in maintaining a body balance, called *homeostasis*. When the balance is upset, problems occur. For example, note the effects when an imbalance occurs in the electrolyte-water balance. Hypertension, congestive heart failure, and a host of other problems ensue. When the balance of blood components is lost, diseases such as leukemia may be diagnosed. The essence of physiology is to assure that the body's functions are maintained in a state of balance. Each body system is governed by principles of physiology.

Basic Physiologic Processes

Three mechanisms are used to move substances (nutrients and wastes) across cell membranes.

1. FILTRATION
    a. depends on differences in pressure on each side of membrane
    b. involves the passage of water and dissolved substances
    c. filters out large materials such as blood proteins, and occurs most often in the capillary network (tiny blood vessels) in the body. Importance to pharmacy: drugs will pass through the blood-brain barrier or into the milk of nursing mothers. (*Note:* The blood-brain barrier refers to the barriers separating the circulating blood from the brain cells and permitting selective passage of certain substances into the brain at specific rates.)
2. DIFFUSION
    a. depends on molecules being in constant motion
    b. results in molecules automatically distributing themselves equally in an available space. For example: Open a bottle of ammonia in a room. Eventually the entire room fills with the permeating smell of ammonia. The molecules have diffused into the air and distributed themselves equally throughout the room.
    c. occurs most readily in our lungs, between the air in the lungs (which contains oxygen and carbon dioxide among other things), and the blood vessels passing through the lungs
    d. is important to pharmacy because inhalers are used to diffuse a drug into the lungs
3. OSMOSIS is a special type of diffusion which relies on a special membrane (called a semipermeable membrane) separating two solutions of unequal concentration. This membrane allows only water to pass. Water will pass from the side having a smaller concentration (fewer particles in the solution) to the side of greater concentration (more particles in the solution) until the concentration of both sides of the semipermeable membrane are equal (that is, the number of particles in the same amount of water on each side of the semipermeable membrane is equal). When equal concentration is achieved, *equilibrium* and *homeostasis* are attained. In pharmacy, drugs can disrupt this equilibrium by introducing particles such as sodium to the body, forcing water to move to the area of greater concentration (more particles). This situation can result in fluid buildup, called edema, or water retention.

    Sodium chloride (salt) is very important to the body system. The concentration of the salt in blood is 0.9% (0.009 Gm. or 9 mg. of salt per every 100 ml. of blood). Changing the concentration elicits an immediate physiologic response to remedy the change by either diluting a higher concentration or making a low concentration more concentrated. In pharmacy, electrolyte concentrations are especially important when dealing with intravenous solutions of various concentrations.

AN OVERVIEW OF ANATOMICAL SYSTEMS

System: Integumentary

Branch of Anatomy: Dermatology

Medical Specialist: Dermatologist

Components

1. Skin
2. Hair
3. Nails
4. Sweat glands
5. Oil glands
6. Hair follicles

Function/Responsibility

- Protects against bacterial invasion
- Maintains proper moisture in tissues
- Regulates body heat and temperature
- Conducts stimuli such as heat, cold, pain, and touch
- Eliminates water and waste products

Additional Information: Sweat glands regulate body temperature by means of water elimination through evaporation. Oil glands (sebaceous glands) keep skin pliable by secreting oils. Hair helps to retain body heat and amplify the sense of touch. Skin color can be indicative of a variety of conditions:

- Bluish (cyanotic)—inadequate supply of oxygen is being transported
- Yellowish (jaundice)—malfunctioning liver
- Paleness (pallor)—indicates possible shock, fright, or anemia
- Redness (flush)—indicates fever

Associated Disorders

Bacterial infections
Fungal infections
Viral infections
Pruritus

An Overview of Anatomical Systems

Dermatitis
Inflammation
Malignancies

Drug Classes/Drugs

Antibiotics: penicillins, tetracyclines, erythromycin, bacitracin, neomycin
Antifungals: amphotericin B, nystatin, clotrimazole, haloprogin, miconazole, tolfanate, zinc undecylanate
Antivirals: acyclovir
Steroids: prednisone, triamcinolone, hydrocortisone
Tranquilizers: diazepam, clordiazepoxide, hydroxyzine
Antihistamines: diphenhydramine, chlorpheniramine, brompheniramine
Antineoplastics: fluorouracil, methotrexate, hydroxyurea

Terms and Definitions

Dermis: deep layer of skin
Desquamation: process by which the dead cell layer is eventually sloughed off and replaced by a new keratin layer
Epidermis: top layer of skin
Intradermal: within the skin
Keratin: layer of dead cells which forms as the outermost part of the epidermis. This layer acts as a protective covering.
Lesions: a structural skin alteration
  a. *Macule:* flat discolored spot, such as a freckle or flat mole
  b. *Papule:* a solid, elevated lesion, such as a pimple
  c. *Nodule:* a palpable solid lesion, such as a cyst
  d. *Vesicle:* a circumscribed elevated lesion, such as a blister
  e. *Pustule:* a superficial, elevated lesion containing pus, such as seen in acne
  f. *Wheal:* an elevated, itching, swollen lesion, such as seen in insect bites
  g. *Telangiectasia:* dilation of superficial blood vessels which form elevated, dark red spots as seen in certain warts
Sebaceous: oil glands
Subcutaneous: subQ or SQ, under the skin

2. **System:** Skeletal

   Branch of Anatomy: Osteology

   Medical Specialist: Orthopedist

Components

1. Bones
2. Ligaments
3. Cartilage
4. Tendons
5. Joints

Function/Responsibility

- Framework of the body
- Support of the body
- Protect vital organs (for example, ribs protect the heart and lungs, the skull protects the brain)
- Store calcium and phosphorous
- Manufacture red blood cells

Additional Information: The body contains a total of 206 bones. The skeleton is divided into the axial skeleton (spine, skull, chest), containing 80 bones, and the appendicular skeleton (upper and lower extremities), which is comprised of 126 bones. Bones serve as a site for attachment for skeletal muscles. The vertebral column (spine) is composed of bones called vertebrae, separated from each other by cartilage pieces called intervertebral discs or "discs." The vertebral column has five sections extending from the neck to the base of the spine:

1. cervical
2. thoracic
3. lumbar
4. sacrum
5. coccyx

Associated Disorders

Arthritis
Gout
Chondrocalcinosis
Bursitis
Osteoarthritis
Paget's Disease (osteities deformans)
Osteoporosis
Osteomyelitis
Bone and joint neoplasms

Drug Classes/Drugs

Analgesics: narcotics (codeine, meperidine), salicylates (aspirin), nonsalicylates (acetaminophen, ibuprofen, propoxyphene)

Gold compounds: gold sodium thiomalate, aurothioglucose
Chelating agents: penicillamine
Nonsteroidal anti-inflammatory agents (NSAIA): indomethacin, naproxen, ibuprofen, fenoprofen, tolmetin, sulindac, phenylbutazone
Steroids: prednisone, hydrocortisone, cortisone
Uricosuric agents: colchicine, allopurinol, probenecid, sulfinpyrazone
Nerve blocking agents: procaine
Muscle relaxants: diazepam
Antihypercalcemic agents: calcitonin
Nutritional agents: calcium
Hormones: estrogen, oxandrolone, testosterone
Antibiotics: methicillin, oxacillin, nafcillin, penicillin, erythromycin, lincomycin, cephalosporins
Immunosuppressive drugs: cyclophosphamide, azathioprine

Terms and Definitions

Appendicular skeleton: skeleton of the arms and legs
Articulations: joints
Axial skeleton: skeleton of the head and trunk
Cartilage: elastic, supporting tissue at joints which protects joints against shock
Cranium: part of skull which encloses the brain
Crepitation: crackling of joints
Crush fractures: fractures which occur without trauma—for example, in osteoporosis, the bones become so weak that the weight of the person alone causes the vertebrae to collapse and crush.
Erythropoiesis: manufacture of red blood cells by red bone marrow
Ligament: tissue structure which holds bones together at their joints
Ossification: bone formation
Osteoarthritis: degenerative joint disease
Sternum: breast bone
Tendons: connective tissue which attaches muscles to bone

3. **System:** Muscular

Branch of Anatomy: Myology

Medical Specialist: Orthopedist

Components

1. Muscles
2. Tendons

Function/Responsibility

- Voluntary movements of body parts (for example, lifting an arm)
- Involuntary movements of body organs (for example, beating of the heart)

Additional Information: There are approximately 656 muscles in the body. Muscle tissue may be categorized as:

1. Involuntary
   a. smooth muscle (nonstriated or visceral muscle)
      (1) digestive tract
      (2) blood vessels
      (3) gallbladder
      (4) urinary bladder
      (5) lungs
   b. cardiac muscle
      (1) heart
2. Voluntary
   a. striated or skeletal muscle
      (1) arms
      (2) legs
      (3) tongue
      (4) abdomen

Associated Disorders

Rheumatism
Myalgia
Spasms
Myositis
Polymyositis
Fibromyositis
Torticollis (wryneck)
Myasthenia gravis
Myotonic myopathies
Drug-induced muscle blocks

Drug Classes/Drugs

Muscle relaxants: diazepam, meprobamate, orphenadrine, quinine
Analgesics: aspirin, acetaminophen

Nerve blocking agents: procaine, lidocaine
Steroids: hydrocortisone, prednisone
Immunosuppressants: methotrexate, cyclophosphamide
Cholinergic drugs: neostigmine, pyridostigmine
Anticonvulsants: phenytoin
Cholinesterase reactivators: pralidoxime
Anticholinergics: atropine
Nutritional supplements: potassium
Nonsteroidal anti-inflammatory agents (NSAIA): indomethacin, naproxen, ibuprofen, fenoprofen, tolmetin, sulindac, phenylbutazone

Terms and Definitions

Atrophy: decreased growth or wasting away
Hypertrophy: increased growth
Intramuscular (IM): within the muscle tissue
Muscle tone: state of continued partial muscle contraction
Rigor mortis: permanent state of muscle contraction after death
Tendons: connective tissue which attaches muscles to bone
Tetany: muscular cramps and twitching caused by a decrease in serum calcium

System: Nervous

Branch of Anatomy: Neurology

Medical Specialist: Neurologist

Components

1. Brain
2. Spinal cord
3. Sense organs
   a. eyes
   b. ears
   c. tongue
   d. nose

Function/Responsibility: Coordinate activities of all the body parts by means of a "stimulus-response" mechanism and a collection of data that is stored in memory.

Additional Information: The brain and spinal cord form the *central nervous system (CNS)*. The sense organs, those structures outside the CNS, comprise the *peripheral nervous system (PNS)*.
Built into the nervous system are two process-oriented nervous systems. The *autonomic nervous system (ANS)* controls involuntary

processes such as breathing and eye-blinking. The *somatic nervous system (SNS)* operates under conscious control and responds only to conscious or voluntary commands to initiate such activities as walking and lifting objects.

The ANS is divided further into the *sympathetic nervous system* and *parasympathetic nervous system*. The sympathetic nervous system, also referred to as "fight and flight," prepares the body for stress or emergency situations by increasing the heart rate, constricting blood vessels, and so on. Generally, the sympathetic nervous system is associated with increased activities.

The parasympathetic nervous system is also known by the phrase, "feed and breed." This part of the nervous system deals primarily with relaxing conditions and a quiet state of the body. The heart rate slows, blood is directed to the stomach for digestion, blood vessels dilate, and so on. The parasympathetic is primarily concerned with digestion and storage of substances required for the body's well-being.

Nerve endings or receptors are specialized. They are affected by specific stimuli. Receptors can be *interoreceptors* (visceral receptors) which are stimulated by sensations from the internal organs or viscera:

1. hunger
2. thirst
3. visceral pain

Proprioreceptors respond to sensations from muscles, tendons, and joints and inform of:

1. position
2. movement
3. deep pressure
4. balance

Exteroreceptors (somatic receptors) are concerned with sensations from outside the body:

1. touch
2. pain
3. temperature
4. vision
5. hearing

The responding motor activities are carried out by structures called *effectors*. Somatic effectors are located in the skeletal muscles and the visceral effectors are found in smooth muscles, cardiac muscle, and secretory glands.

Nerve pathways are connected by junctions called *synapses*. In order for nerve impulses to cross a synapse, chemical substances called neurotransmitters are required to carry the impulse. The neurotransmitters are specific for the type of response elicited:

1. excitatory neurotransmitters
   a. acetylcholine (Ach)
   b. epinephrine (Epi)
2. inhibitory neurotransmitter
   a. gamma-aminobutyric acid (GABA)

Associated Disorders

Pain
Cephalalgia (headache)
Trigeminal neuralgia
Vertigo
Seizure disorders
Narcolepsy
Bacterial meningitis
Mycotic meningitis
Brain abscess
Multiple sclerosis
Tremors
Parkinsonism
Ballism
Hemiballism
Huntington's chorea

Drug Classes/Drugs

Analgesics: aspirin (ASA), acetaminophen (APAP), propoxyphene
Narcotic analgesics: codeine, meperidine, hydromorphone, methadone
Anticonvulsants: carbamazepine, phenytoin, primidone
Tranquilizers: chlorpromazine, meprobamate, diazepam, haloperidol
Sedatives: phenobarbital
Antiemetics: perphenazine, meclizine, dimenhydrinate
Stimulants: amphetamine, ephedrine, dextroamphetamine, methylphenidate
Antibiotics: chloramphenicol, penicillin G, ampicillin, kanamycin, gentamicin, carbenicillin, tetracycline
Antifungals: amphotericin B
Steroids: dexamethasone, prednisone
Antiparkinson agents: levodopa, carbidopa

Terms and Definitions

Afferent nerve cells: transmit sensory impulses to CNS
Axons: part of nerve cell that carries impulses away from the cell
Connector nerve cells (interneurons): transmit impulses between afferent and efferent neurons
Dendrites: branches of a nerve cell; carry impulses to the nerve cell
Efferent nerve cells: transmit motor impulses away from CNS
Gustatory: refers to the sense of taste
Learning: a process by which the nervous system collects and stores information received from experiences
Neurons: the nerve cell
Neurotransmitters: chemical substances which facilitate the transmission of impulses across synapses
Olfactory: refers to the sense of smell
Ophthalmic: refers to the eye
Optic: refers to the sense of sight
Otic: refers to the sense of hearing
Synapse: junction between two neurons
Tactile: refers to the sense of touch

5. **System: Cardiovascular/Circulatory**

Branch of Anatomy: Cardiology (heart), Hematology (blood)

Medical Specialist: Cardiologist (heart), Vascular Surgeon (blood vessels), Hematologist (blood)

Components:

1. Heart
2. Blood vessels
3. Lymph vessels
4. Lymph nodes
5. Spleen
6. Blood

Function/Responsibility: Supplies the cells of the body with oxygen and nutrients, transports chemical body regulators (hormones), produces and transports body defenses (antibodies), transports cellular waste products for elimination, and regulates body temperature.

Additional Information: The heart pumps blood through two main pathways in the body. The pulmonary circuit carries blood from the heart to the lungs by way of pulmonary veins and from the lungs back to the heart via pulmonary arteries. The much larger systemic circuit carries blood throughout the body by means of arteries which carry blood away from the heart, to capillaries throughout the body and finally back to the heart by way of veins.

The lymph system passes lymph fluid through spaces between cells. This lymph fluid is filtered through lymph nodes, filtering out bacteria and other foreign particles, before emptying into veins.

The spleen is composed largely of the same material which makes up lymph nodes. The spleen filters out old, worn-out red blood cells and extracts the iron from them to be reused by bone marrow to make new red blood cells. Although the spleen has an important function, it is not essential to life.

Blood is composed of a liquid part and solid components. The liquid is called *plasma* and the solid elements consist of red blood cells, white blood cells, and platelets.

Arterial blood pressure (BP) measurement is the result of two readings using a blood pressure device called a *sphygmomanometer*. The reading is displayed as the systolic reading over the diastolic reading. The systolic reading is a measure of the force of blood pushing against arterial blood vessel walls when the ventricles (lower chambers of the heart) are contracting. The diastolic reading represents the force of blood pushing against the arteries when the ventricles are relaxed. Variations from normal blood pressure may indicate hypertension, heart disease, or hardening of the arteries. The average normal blood pressure varies with age. For example, the young adult male has an average BP of 120/80 (systolic/diastolic).

Associated Disorders

Anemia
Vitamin B-12 deficiency
Vitamin deficiencies
Allergic reactions
Leukemia
Coagulation disorders
Disseminated intravascular coagulation
Lymphoma (Hodgkin's Disease)
Hypertension
Shock
Congestive heart failure (CHF)
Tachycardia
Bradycardia
Hypertensive Cardiovascular Disease
Angina pectoris
Myocardial infarction (MI)
Bacterial endocarditis
Cardiovascular syphilis
Raynaud's disease
Phlebitis

Drug Classes/Drugs

Iron preparations: ferrous sulfate, ferrous gluconate
Vitamin B-12 preparations: cyanocobalamine, liver extract
Vitamin preparations: pyridoxine, thiamine, folic acid
Vitamin K preparations: phytonadione
Antihistamines: diphenhydramine
Steroids: dexamethasone, prednisone
Sympathomimetics: epinephrine
Antineoplastic agents: chlorambucil, cyclophosphamide, melphalan, vincristine, mechlorethamine, procarbazine, doxorubicin, bleomycin
Anticoagulants: heparin
Diuretics: hydrochlorothiazide, furosemide, spironolactone, triamterene
Antihypertensive agents (hypotensive agents): methyldopa, clonidine, reserpine, hydralazine, guanethidine
Vasopressors: isoproterenol, dopamine, metaraminol, levarterenol (norepinephrine)
Cardiac agents: digoxin, digitalis, digitoxin, nitroglycerin
Electrolyte replacements: potassium, potassium chloride
Beta-blocking agents: propranolol, metoprolol
Antiarrhythmic agents: procainamide, quinidine
Antibiotics: penicillin, tetracycline, erythromycin, methicillin, streptomycin, nafcillin
Vasodilators: nylidrin, isoxsuprine, papaverine, tolazoline

Terms and Definitions

Arteries: blood vessels which carry blood away from the heart
Capillaries: networks of minute blood vessels which connect arteries and veins
CBC: complete blood count, an analysis of RBCs, WBCs, and platelets
Differential white count: "differential" is a test used to count the amount of each type of white blood cell making up the total leukocyte (WBC) count
Edema: collection of fluid in body tissues
Embolus: a thrombus, blood clot, that breaks free and flows in a blood vessel
Erythropoiesis: process of forming RBCs
Hemoglobin: an iron-containing pigment in the red blood cell which carries oxygen in the blood
Hemostasis: the blood clotting mechanism
Hgb: hemoglobin

Platelets: an element in blood important in the clotting process of blood, thrombocytes (old term)

RBC: red blood cell, erythrocyte, carries oxygen

Serum: fluid portion of blood resulting after blood clots

Thrombus: abnormal clot that develops in a blood vessel

Veins: blood vessels which carry blood away from the heart

WBC: white blood cell, leukocyte, used in defense against infection

6. **System: Respiratory/Pulmonary**

Branch of Anatomy: Pulmonary

Medical Specialist: Pulmonologist

Components

1. Nose
2. Pharynx
3. Larynx
4. Trachea
5. Bronchi
6. Lungs
7. Sinuses

Function/Responsibility: Supplies oxygen to the blood (oxygenation of the blood) and removes the carbon dioxide (a waste product resulting from metabolism).

Additional Information: When you breathe, air passes through the nostrils, where it is moistened, warmed, and filtered through nasal hairs on its way to the lungs. Once inhaled, the air in the lungs is extracted of its oxygen portion which is transported into the blood (attaches to the RBC in blood) for use by the cells. Carbon dioxide, a waste product of metabolism, is diffused into the air sac in the lung and exhaled out into the atmosphere.

The breathing activity is also responsible for speech production or phonation. The breathing process forces air from the lungs through the larynx upon exhaling, thereby producing sounds.

The lungs are referred to as lobes. Sections of the lung have definite locations:

1. left upper lobe
2. left lower lobe
3. right upper lobe
4. right middle lobe
5. right lower lobe

Associated Disorders

Upper respiratory infection (URI)
Sinusitis
Rhinitis
Bronchitis
Asthma
Bronchiectasis
Lower respiratory infection
Pneumonia
Tuberculosis
Emphysema
Pleurisy

Drug Classes/Drugs

Analgesics: aspirin, acetaminophen
Antipyretics: aspirin
Antihistamines: diphenhydramine, chlorpheniramine, brompheniramine
Vasoconstrictors: phenylephrine, naphazoline, ephedrine, pseudoephedrine
Antitussives: hydrocodone, dextromethorphan, codeine
Antibiotics: penicillin, ampicillin, amoxicillin, erythromycin, tetracycline
Steroids: hydrocortisone, prednisone
Bronchodilator: theophylline, aminophylline, isoproterenol, epinephrine
Antitubercular agents: isoniazid, ethambutol, ethionamide, pyrazinamide, rifampin

Terms and Definitions

Alveolar ducts: tubes which carry air to the alveolar sacs
Alveolar sacs: air sacs found within the lungs
Apex: top of the lung
Apnea: breathing stops
Base: bottom of the lung
Breathing: the mechanical act of inhaling and exhaling
Bronchi: two branches of the trachea, each one extending into a lung.
Bronchial tree: the air passageways consisting of a large tube, the trachea, and dividing into smaller passageways, called the bronchi, which divide into even smaller passageways called the bronchioles
Bronchioles: smaller divisions of the bronchi in the lungs

Dyspnea: labored or difficult breathing

Hypoxia: deficiency in the amount or utilization of oxygen by body tissues

Larynx: voice box

Metabolism: physical and chemical changes which nutrients undergo in order to become usable by the body

Pharynx: throat

Respiration: refers to the process of exchanging oxygen and carbon dioxide between body cells and the cell surroundings. Oxygen is transported to the cells, while carbon dioxide is transported away from the cells and out to the atmosphere.

Trachea: windpipe

System: Digestive

Branch of Anatomy: Gastroenterology

Medical Specialist: Gastroenterologist

Components

1. Mouth
2. Tongue
3. Teeth
4. Pharynx
5. Esophagus
6. Stomach
7. Small intestine
8. Large intestine
9. Accessory glands
   a. salivary glands
   b. liver
   c. gallbladder
   d. pancreas

Function/Responsibility: Food which has been consumed is converted into a form which can be used by the body cells for growth, energy, and repair.

Additional Information: Of all the systems comprising the human anatomy, the digestive system has the most profound effect on drugs consumed orally.

Drugs are sensitive to acid/base balance. In order for drugs to achieve their intended effect, the acidity of the stomach and alkalinity are considered.

The intestines contain bacterial and yeast organisms called "flora," which keep each other in balance. An overgrowth of one or the other produces severe health complications.

The liver is a vital organ. It is responsible for controlling blood sugar levels, storing a reserve of nutrients (glycogen), producing blood clotting factors (prothrombin and fibrinogen), producing bile salts used to digest fat and aid in the absorption of vitamin K from the gastrointestinal (GI) tract, and detoxifying many substances, including drugs.

Food is composed of starches and sugars (collectively called carbohydrates), fats, and proteins. The digestive process breaks these complex compounds into their simplest elements:

1. starches and sugars to monosaccharides
2. proteins to amino acids
3. fats to fatty acids and glycerol

The acid found in the stomach is "hydrochloric acid" (HCl). This acid is responsible for facilitating the action of digestive enzymes on the food entering the stomach.

Digestion of food begins in the mouth when the digestive enzyme, ptyalin, breaks down starch. The mouth is also responsible for mechanical digestion, called mastication (chewing). Absorption of digested food begins in the stomach to some degree, but almost all absorption occurs from the small intestinal walls.

Associated Disorders

Nausea and vomiting (often considered symptoms)
Hiccups (singultus)
Constipation
Gastrointestinal gas (flatulence)
Diarrhea
Candidiasis
Oral cancer
Glossitis
Leukoplakia
Reflux Esophagitis
Gastritis
Peptic ulcer
Gastric ulcer
Duodenal ulcer
Jegunal ulcer
Stomach carcinoma
Enteritis
Colitis
Sprue
Jaundice
Hepatitis
Cirrhosis

Cholecystitis
Cholelithiasis (gallstones)
Pancreatitis
Peritonitis

Drug Classes/Drugs

Antihistamines: dimenhydrinate

Antiemetics: prochlorperazine (phenothiazine)

Tranquilizers: prochlorperazine, metoclopramide

Sedatives: pentobarbital

Local anesthetics: viscous lidocaine

Antispasmodics: atropine sulfate

Laxatives: docusate sodium, cascara sagrada, bisacodyl, phenolphthalein, psyllium hydrophilic mucilloid, milk of magnesia, citrate of magnesia, lactulose

Antiflatulence medications: simethicone

Antidiarrheal agents: diphenoxylate with atropine, loperamide, paregoric

Analgesics: pentazocine, meperidine

Antimicrobials: ampicillin, clindamycin, "aminoglycosides," metronidazole, sulfasalazine, tetracycline, trimethoprim-sulfamethoxazole

Antifungal agents: nystatin, clotrimazole, ketoconazole

Antacids: aluminum hydroxide, magnesium hydroxide, magnesium carbonate, magnesium trisilicate, alginic acid

Histamine H_2-receptor blockers: cimetidine, ranitidine

Cholinergic agents: bethanechol chloride

Gastrointestinal stimulants: metaclopramide

Antiulcer agents: sucralfate

Antineoplastic agents: mitomycin C, 5-fluorouracil, adriamycin, cytarabine

Steroids: prednisone, cortisol, hydrocortisone

Diuretics: spironolactone, furosemide

Pancreatic supplements: trade name products; Cotazyme, Festal, Viokase, Ilozyme

Miscellaneous: chenodeoxycholic acid (dissolves some cholesterol stones)

Terms and Definitions

Absorption: passage of food from the digestive tract to the blood after the food has been broken down during the process of digestion

Anabolism: constructive metabolism or buildup of simple substances synthesized into complex substances which are used for body/protein rebuilding

Basal metabolic rate (BMR): the amount of energy used for metabolism when a body is at rest

Calories: measurement of the quantity of heat required to raise one gram of water, one degree Celsius (centigrade). This unit is used to express the heat output of an organism or energy value given off by food.

Catabolism: destructive metabolism or breakdown of complex organic substances to simpler substances with energy being released

Defecation: elimination of feces from the rectum

Digestion: process of chemically breaking down complex food material into soluble material which can be absorbed by the body

Duodenum: the tube leading from the stomach to the small intestine; it is the first of three portions of the small intestine.

Electrolytes: a substance such as sodium or chloride which is capable of carrying an electrical charge

Esophagus: a collapsible tube which opens into the stomach

Feces: waste product resulting from digestion of food

Gallstones: hard, stone-like masses formed in the gallbladder

Insulin: a hormone produced by the pancreas, responsible for the breakdown of sugar

Metabolism: the total chemical processes of anabolism and catabolism

Minerals: inorganic chemical compounds required by body processes for appropriate functioning

Occult blood: blood, abnormally found in the stools

Peristalsis: wave-like movements resulting from contraction and relaxation of muscles, especially in the intestines

Pharynx: a passageway common to both the respiratory and digestive systems

Vitamins: group of organic compounds required for normal metabolism, growth, and maintenance of life in man

System: Endocrine

Branch of Anatomy: Endocrinology

Medical Specialist: Endocrinologist

Components

1. Glands
   a. pituitary
   b. thyroid
   c. parathyroid
   d. pancreas
   e. adrenal

An Overview of Anatomical Systems

        f. gonads
           (1) testicles
           (2) ovaries
        g. thymus
    2. Hormones

Function/Responsibility: Chemical control, unification and coordination of the many complex activities of the whole body.

Additional Information: Saliva, mucus, and pancreatic juice secretions produced by specific glands called *exocrine glands* are carried by tubes called ducts. *Endocrine glands* are ductless and pass their secretions, called *hormones*, directly into the blood. The blood circulation transports hormones to their target organs.

Both the endocrine and nervous systems control bodily functions. The effects of the endocrine system (via chemical mediators) take longer. The effects of the endocrine activities last longer than the effects of the nervous system, which uses electrical impulses.

Only minute amounts of hormones are required to elicit a physiological response. Hormones function to regulate the rate of existing body processes. Hormones do not initiate a process. Hormones may be associated with either metabolism or regulatory functions. For instance, insulin is a metabolism hormone concerned with carbohydrate metabolism. The thyroid hormone (thyroxin) regulates the body's basal metabolic rate. Neither hormone initiates either process.

A third group of hormones have a *morphogenetic* function. These hormones influence the development and growth of body tissues or specific organs. Morphogenetic hormones are represented by growth hormones (secreted by the pituitary) and estrogens, which exert their influence on the uterus and vagina.

The adrenal glands, situated above the kidneys, produce hormones called *steroids*. These steroids are divided into glucocorticoids (sugar hormones) and mineralocorticoids (salt hormones). Glucocorticoids exert their function by regulating glucose metabolism. Mineralocorticoids assure that a balance between various minerals (especially sodium and potassium) is maintained to regulate the body's water content.

The adrenal glands also secrete epinephrine (adrenalin) and norepinephrine (noradrenalin), which increase the heart rate and the beating strength of the heart, and raise blood pressure by constricting blood vessels.

The pancreas is located behind the stomach and is the gland responsible for secreting the insulin hormone and digestive juices. Insulin is produced by the beta cells in the pancreas. Drugs such as tolbutamide and tolazamide are used to stimulate insulin production in failing and defective beta cells.

Refer to Table 4-1 for a summary of endocrine functions.

TABLE 4-1

Endocrine Glands and Their Functions

Gland	Hormone Secretion	Function	Noteworthy
PITUITARY	growth hormone (GH)	stimulates the rate of cell growth	The pituitary gland is also known as the hypophysis and sometimes referred to as the master gland.
	adrenocorticotropic hormone (ACTH)	stimulates the adrenal gland to produce glucocorticoids	
	thyrotropic hormone (TSH)	stimulates the thyroid to release its hormone called thyroxin	
	follicle-stimulating hormone (FSH)	stimulates the growth of follicle cells surrounding the ovum (female egg cell)	
	germinal-stimulating hormones (GSH)	stimulate cells in the testes to produce sperm	
	leutenizing hormone (LH)	responsible for ovulation in the female (release of a mature egg cell from the ovary)	
	interstitial cell-stimulating hormone (ICSH)	stimulates cells in testes to produce testosterone	
	luteotropic hormone (LTH or prolactin)	responsible for the growth of the breast tissue and milk production in pregnant females	
	melanocyte-stimulating hormone (MSH)	stimulates cells in the skin responsible for pigment production	
	vasopressin (pitressin), antidiuretic hormone (ADH)	responsible for the constriction of coronary arteries, reduction of cardiac output, reduction of urine output	
	oxytocin (pitocin)	acts on the smooth muscle of the uterus during pregnancy by stimulating contractions near the time of child delivery, controls bleeding after delivery, stimualtes milk production for nursing	
THYROID	thyroid hormone (thyroxin)	stimulates metabolism of all body cells (increases basal metabolic rate—BMR)	The thyroid promotes the growth and ossification of bones and the development of teeth.
PARATHYROID	parathyroid hormone	regulates calcium and phosphorous metabolism	
PANCREAS	insulin	increases the rate of glucose metabolism, decreases amount of glucose in blood, increases amount of glycogen stored in the tissues (for example, liver)	
	glucagon	stimulates liver to break down stored glycogen into glucose	

TABLE 4-1 (Continued)

Gland	Hormone Secretion	Function	Noteworthy
ADRENALS (medulla portion)	epinephrine (adrenalin)	stimulates constriction of skin blood vessels, pupil dilation, piloerection, intestinal muscle relaxation, dilation of skeletal muscle blood vessels, bronchodilation, increase in heart muscle contraction	This gland is also referred to as *suprarenal glands*.
	norepinephrine (noradrenalin)	stimulates constriction of skin blood vessels, pupil dilation, piloerection, intestinal muscle relaxation, increase in heart muscle contraction	
ADRENALS (cortex portion)	cortical hormones glucocorticoids (cortisol, corticosterone)	stimulates gluconeogenesis by the liver, decrease protein stores in body cells, fat storage and metabolism	As a group, the cortical steroids are called corticosteroids (primarily composed of cortisol, corticosterone, and aldosterone).
	mineralocorticoids (aldosterone)	stimulates the increase reabsorption of sodium by the kidneys, decrease reabsorption of potassium by the kidneys, exchange of sodium transfer into cells while transporting potassium out of cells, and controls water balance in the body	
GONADS	androgens (male hormone) testosterone	responsible for normal growth, development, and functioning of male reproductive organs and sex characteristics (for example, voice, beard growth, muscle tone), stimulates bone growth	In the male, the gonad is called the testes. In the female, the gonad is called the ovaries.
	estrogens (female hormones) estradiol	inhibit FSH stimulation, induces ovulation, stimulates growth of uterus, uterine tubes, and mammary ducts, development of sex characteristics (for example, voice, fat deposit)	
	progesterone	prepares uterus for implantation of fertilized egg cell, inhibits ovulation during pregnancy	Progesterone is sometimes called the "pregnancy hormone."
THYMUS	"hormone-like" factor	stimulates spleen and lymph nodes to produce lymphocytes	The thymus shrinks with age until it nearly disappears in adulthood. Actual endocrine functions are unknown.

Associated Disorders

Panhypopituitarism
Hypopituitary cachexia
Diabetes insipidus
Diabetes mellitus
Simple goiter
Hypothyroidism
Hyperthyroidism
Thyroid cancer
Thyroiditis
Hypoparathyroidism
Hyperparathyroidism
Osteomalacia
Osteoporosis
Paget's Disease (osteitis deformans)
Prostatitis
Pancreatitis
Adrenocortical insufficiency
Adrenocortical overactivity (Cushing's Syndrome)
Male hypogonadism and hypergonadism
Female hypogonadism and hypergonadism
Amenorrhea

Drug Classes/Drugs

Steroids: hydrocortisone, prednisone, cortisone, desoxycorticosterone, fludrocortisone
Sex hormones: testosterone, diethylstilbesterol, ethinylestradiol, conjugated estrogens
Fertility drugs: bromocriptine, clomiphene
Hormones: vasopressin, calcitonin, insulin
Diuretics: hydrochlorothiazide, furosemide, ethacrynic acid
Thyroid agents: thyroid extract, levothyroxine, iodine, propylthiouracil (PTU), methimazole, liothyronine, liotrix
Chemotherapeutic agents: doxorubicin
Electrolyte replacement/supplement therapy: calcium gluconate, calcium chloride, calcium carbonate, calcium lactate
Vitamin therapy: dihydrotachysterol (vitamin D), dihydroxycholecalciferol, calciferol
Antidiabetic agents: tolbutamide, chlorpropamide, tolazamide, glyburide, acetohexamide, glipizide

Terms and Definitions

Adrenocorticotropic hormone (ACTH): secreted by the pituitary, this hormone is responsible for stimulating the adrenal glands to increase the production of glucocorticoids (hormone which affects the metabolism of glucose).

Androgens: male hormones

Antidiuretic hormone (ADH): a pituitary hormone responsible for the reduction of urine by increasing reabsorption of water by the kidney. Also known as vasopressin, pitressin, or pituitrin, this hormone causes the constriction of coronary arteries in the heart, and reduces the cardiac output by lessening the strength of the heart muscle.

Glands: structures in the body which produce secretions such as saliva, pancreatic juice, and hormones

Gluconeogenesis: formation of glucose by the liver from noncarbohydrate sources

Glycogenolysis: breakdown of glycogen from a complex carbohydrate to monosaccharides such as glucose

Goiter: enlargement of the thyroid gland as a result of a gland disorder

Gonads: sex glands

Growth hormone (GH): hormone secreted by the pituitary gland and functions to increase the rate of growth of all body cells

Hormones: chemical substances produced by specific organs; these chemicals have specific regulatory effects on body functions.

Hypophysis: pituitary gland

Insulin: hormone secreted by pancreas and used to decrease the blood sugar level

Ossification: process of hardening into bone

Oxytocin: a hormone secreted by the pituitary, responsible for producing powerful contractions in the uterus

Piloerection: hairs "stand on end"

System: Male Reproductive

Branch of Anatomy: Genitourinary

Medical Specialist: Urologist

Components

1. Testes
2. Scrotum
3. Penis

4. Accessory organs
   a. ducts
      (1) duct of epididymis
      (2) ductus deferens
      (3) ejaculatory ducts
   b. urethra
5. Glands
   a. seminal vesicles
   b. prostate gland
   c. bulbourethral glands
6. Semen

Function/Responsibility: The male reproductive organ is responsible for the perpetuation of the human species through sexual reproduction. In addition, the male reproductive organ produces hormones which assure the development of male characteristics.

Additional Information: The male reproductive organ includes two testes. These testes produce spermatozoa and male hormones.

Semen, the reproductive fluid of the male, contains spermatozoa plus fluid from the seminal vesicles, prostate gland, and bulbourethral glands. The penis is the male organ which conveys the reproductive fluid from the male into the female. The ejaculation of fluid from the penis contains from 200 to 400 million sperm cells, maintaining a fertilizing vitality lasting twenty-four to seventy-two hours.

Associated Disorders

Gonorrhea
Syphilis
Urethritis
Balanoposthitis
Balanitis
Lymphogranulomas

Drug Classes/Drugs

Antibiotics: penicillin, ampicillin, amoxicillin, tetracycline, sulfonamides (for example, Gantrisin), streptomycin

Terms and Definitions

Circumcision: surgical removal of a free fold of skin (prepuce) along the base of the end of the penis

Cowper's glands: bulbourethral glands responsible for producing an alkaline fluid which helps to neutralize the acidity of the fluid produced by the prostate gland

Ejaculation: expulsion of semen from the male through the penis

Genitalia: sex organs (male—penis; female—vagina)

Scrotum: sac containing the testes

Semen: reproductive fluid

Spermatic cord: collective term for the ducts, blood vessels, nerves, lymphatics, and tissue coverings ascending from the testes and passing out of the scrotum

Spermatogenesis: production of spermatozoa

Spermatozoa: male sex cells

10. **System: Female Reproductive**

Branch of Anatomy: Gynecology

Medical Specialist: Gynecologist

Components

1. Ovary (gonad)
2. Accessory organs
   a. uterus
   b. uterine tubes (oviducts)
   c. vagina
3. Vulva (genitalia)
4. Mammary glands
5. Menstrual cycle

Function/Responsibility: The female reproductive system is responsible for the perpetuation of the human species through sexual reproduction. In addition, the female reproductive organs produce hormones which assure the development of female characteristics.

Additional Information: The vagina provides the passageway for the fetus during birth and provides the outlet for the excretion of the menstrual flow. It is also the receptive organ for the penis.

The menstrual cycle is usually completed every twenty-eight days, but may vary in normal healthy women. The blood flow during menses occurs during the last five days of the cycle. Approximately ten days after the menstrual flow stops, an ovum is discharged. This process is known as ovulation.

The areola surrounding the nipple darkens in color during pregnancy.

Spermatozoa are viable in the female reproductive tract for at least forty-eight hours.

Emotional disturbances can cause irregularities in the menstrual cycle.

Menstruation stops during pregnancy.

Menopause usually begins between ages forty-five and fifty. During menopause, reproductive glands have a reduction in secretions, the ovaries atrophy (as do the uterus and other sex organs), and physical and psychological disturbances are usually characterized by hot flushes, headaches, sweating, dizzy spells, worry, fear, and irritability.

Associated Disorders

Gonorrhea
Syphilis
Trichomoniasis
Candidiasis
Urethritis
Lymphogranulomas
Dyspareunia
Infertility
Amenorrhea
Uterine bleeding
Endometriosis
Vulvitis
Salpingitis (pelvic inflammatory disease—PID)
Premenstrual tension
Primary or functional dysmenorrhea
Carcinoma of the breast

Drug Classes/Drugs

Antibiotics: penicillin, ampicillin, amoxicillin, tetracycline, streptomycin, kanamycin
Antiprotozoan: metronidazole
Antifungal: nystatin
Analgesics: aspirin, acetaminophen, codeine, pentazocine
Topical anesthetics: dibucaine, lidocaine
Sedative: phenobarbital
Fertility drugs: clomiphene
Hormones: ethinyl estradiol, medroxyprogesterone, conjugated estrogens, estrogen-progestin combinations, testosterone
Antihistamines: diphenhydramine, tripelennamine
Tranquilizers: diazepam
Diuretics: hydrochlorothiazide
Nonsteroidal anti-inflammatory agents (NSAIA): naproxen, ibuprofen
Steroids: prednisone
Nonsteroidal estrogen antagonist: tamoxifen
Cytotoxic chemotherapeutic agents: 5-fluorouracil, cyclophosphamide, methotrexate, chlorambucil, vincristine, doxorubicin, melphalan

Terms and Definitions

Areola: pigmented area around the nipple on the breast
Cervix: the constricted lower end of the uterus

Endometrium: mucous membrane lining the uterus

Fallopian tubes: ovarian tubes, uterine tubes

Fertilization: the union of the male's sperm with the female's egg

Gestation: pregnancy

Hymen: a fold of mucous membrane that partially covers the posterior portion of the entrance to the vagina

Mammary glands: breasts

Menopause: the phase of a woman's life when menstruation ceases

Menstruation: the cyclical discharge of bloody fluid from the uterus which occurs between puberty and menopause

Ovulation: eggs become mature and are shed from the ovary on a specific schedule called a menstrual cycle

Placenta: organ to which the fetus is attached by means of the umbilical cord and which supplies nourishment to the fetus while removing waste products

Arithmetic Review

Specific skills are needed for every occupation. An individual completing the tasks required by the job should be proficient in those skills if he or she is going to perform the activity properly. Pharmacy technology requires a proficiency in mathematical procedures, concepts, and numbers manipulation. Pharmacy calculations is a title given to a fundamental tool required in pharmacy. The importance of mathematics and calculations cannot be stressed enough.

At one point, the importance of calculations in pharmacy was questionable. Drug companies manufactured drugs in prescribed dosages and forms (liquids, tablets, capsules, suppositories, etc.). The compounding of medications that was required in the past diminished. "Old-time" physicians who prescribed their specially compounded remedies and potions became fewer and fewer.

However, as drugs became more potent and the state of the art of pharmacy progressed, pharmacy calculations ironically became even more critical. Potent drugs required tailored dosage calculations based on body weight, body surface area, age, and laboratory test results. The gap between therapeutic drug levels (the level at which research shows a drug to provide an effect that has a positive outcome) and toxic levels (levels which can cause harm in an individual) narrowed. The role of calculations as a tool in pharmacy took on renewed emphasis. Specific calculations for antibiotics, newborn intensive care units, intravenous admixtures, and hyperalimentation supported and demanded the need for proficiency in pharmaceutical calculations. It follows, therefore, that you should be thoroughly acquainted with basic arithmetic operations, fundamental mathematical concepts (decimals, percentages, ratio and proportion), and simple algebraic procedures.

Decimals

This text presumes that you have a basic knowledge of mathematics and its operations. However, this chapter is designed to refresh those mathematical skills in areas that specifically involve pharmacy and its computations. Once the review of decimals, percentages, and ratio/proportion is completed, you will see how to apply this knowledge to problems reflecting contemporary pharmacy practice. Many of these problems are derived from actual Physician's Orders and prescriptions.

Consult a basic arithmetic and math text to sharpen those rarely used fundamental skills in math which are especially important to those operations involving pharmacy practice. A basic knowledge in pharmacy calculations will enable you to handle the array of calculations customarily associated with pharmacy.

DECIMALS

Can you complete the following problems?

1. Convert 0.30 to a fraction.
2. Convert $\frac{1}{4}$ to a decimal.
3. Add 0.260 + 1.9 + 4.32 + 2
4. Multiply 4.9 by 2.3876
5. Divide 11.49 by 3.83
6. Subtract 6.72 from 12.9

Were your answers as follows?

1. $\frac{3}{10}$
2. 0.25
3. 8.48
4. 11.69924
5. 3.0
6. 6.18

If you got these answers, you should have no difficulty with decimals. However, if you were not too successful, this chapter should refresh some decimal operations that perhaps have been forgotten.

A decimal is a way to express fractions ($\frac{1}{4}$, $\frac{1}{2}$, $\frac{30}{72}$, etc.) as whole numbers. It is much easier to work with numbers in a decimal notation than it is to work with numbers expressed as fractions. Pharmacy drug measurements are often expressed in amounts less than 1. These measurements can be indicated in fractional notation. In many instances they are so noted. For example, you may see bottles of phenobarbital (a sedative drug) expressed in strengths of $\frac{1}{4}$ gr. and $\frac{1}{2}$ gr.; nitroglycerine (a heart medication used for angina) as $\frac{1}{100}$ gr., $\frac{1}{150}$ gr., $\frac{1}{200}$ gr.; thyroid extract (a drug used for an underactive thyroid) as $\frac{1}{4}$ gr., $\frac{1}{2}$ gr., and so on. In order to make the process of calculating amounts for specific compounding orders or special prescription requests, it is much easier to convert fractions to their decimal notations (that is, $\frac{1}{4} = 0.25$, $\frac{1}{2} = 0.50$, $\frac{3}{8} = 0.375$, etc.). In the decimal form, numbers are treated as whole numbers, with the only difference being the position of the decimal point.

There are a number of rules to follow when working with decimals.

Rule. Pay close attention to the position of the decimal point. When adding and subtracting decimal numbers, be sure that the decimal points are lined up. The decimal point must also be lined up in the answer.

The RIGHT Way:	The WRONG Way:
1.2345	1.2345
12.3456	12.3456
1234.56	1234.56
7	7
0.3456	0.3456

Rule. In the multiplication of decimals, the sum of the number of figures to the right of the decimal point in the multiplicand and multiplier equals the number of places after the decimal point in the resulting product.

Example:

(multiplicand)	2.57	(two numbers follow the decimal point)
(multiplier)	× 3.4	(one number follows the decimal point)
(product)	8.738	(three figures follow the decimal point. This represents the sum of the numbers following the decimal point in the multiplicand and the multiplier)

Rule. In division of decimals, move the decimal point in the divisor to the right until the number becomes a whole number. Keep count of the number of times you moved the decimal point. Move the decimal point the same number of places in the dividend.

Example:

$$\text{divisor}\overline{)\text{dividend}}^{\text{quotient}} \quad \text{or} \quad \text{dividend/divisor} = \text{quotient}$$

$$679.684/14.63$$

Moving the decimal point two places to the right changes the decimal-fraction divisor, 14.63, to a *whole* number, 1463. Following the rule, move the decimal point in the dividend two places to the right. The dividend is now changed from 679.684 to 67968.4.

Be sure the decimal point is lined up in the quotient directly above the decimal point in the dividend. Complete the division operation. The answer (the quotient) should read: 46.4.

The final division process leaves you with a remainder of 582. How do you treat this remainder? You can complete the problem in a variety of ways.

1. If the remainder is greater than one-half of the divisor, increase the last digit in the quotient by 1. Note, therefore, that the remainder of 582 is more than $\frac{1}{2}$ of the divisor (that is, 582/1463 = 0.58). (*Note:* $\frac{1}{2}$ = 0.5, therefore, 0.58 is greater than $\frac{1}{2}$.) You have an option of making the resulting quotient 46.5. This is referred to as "rounding."
2. Another option is to add zeros after the last digit in the dividend without changing the numerical value of the dividend (67968.4 = 67968.40 = 67968.400, etc.). The number of places you want to carry a number after the decimal point will determine the number of zeros you must add on to the dividend. For instance, if you want to carry the number to three decimal places, you would add two zeros to the dividend, thereby making three places after the decimal point. The division process continues with the following result:

$$67968.400/1463 = 46.458$$

Again, after completing the division, you find that you still have a remainder of 346, which is less than one-half of the divisor. You may drop this remainder and leave the quotient at 46.458.

There may be times which warrant "rounding off." In the previous example, you may want to reduce the number of places beyond the decimal to fewer than you have currently chosen. If you want to take your answer to two places beyond the decimal point, your quotient would read 46.46 (that is, rounding 46.458, the last digit, 8, is greater than 5, which permits you to increase the number to the left of the 8 by one digit, or in this case, the 5 becomes a 6). If you were to take the number to only one place beyond the decimal point, you would follow the same procedure. The quotient, 46.458 becomes 46.46, which when rounded to the ones place beyond the decimal point becomes 46.5 (the last 6 in 46.46 being greater than 5 enables you to increase the 4 after the decimal point to 5, resulting in the final quotient of 46.5).

Note: The magic number of 5 is not magic at all. The decimal (from the French meaning "tenth") system is based on 10, which is also the basis for the metric system. Therefore, the halfway point from 1 to 10 is 5. Any number greater than 5 is obviously more than half. A final note to remember is the rule of rounding when your remainder is 5 or a 5 follows the digit you want to round up or down. If the number to be rounded is an odd number followed by 5, round up the odd number by 1. If the number to be rounded is an even number followed by 5, the even number remains unchanged.

There are times when it is necessary to convert fractions to decimals. This is done simply by dividing the numerator by the denominator. For example, the fraction $\frac{1}{4}$ is converted to a decimal by dividing the numerator (top number) by the denominator (bottom number).

$$4\overline{)1.000}\begin{array}{c}0.250\end{array}0.250 = \text{decimal fraction } \tfrac{1}{4}$$

It is a good practice to hold a position to the left of a decimal point with a zero if there is no whole number, such as in the preceding example. It is quite easy to leave the number as .250 with no whole number to the left of the decimal. Identifying this position with a zero does not change the value of the number and has the benefit of preventing potential errors caused by inadvertent markings or incorrect placement of the decimal point.

Convert the following fractions to decimal numbers:

$$\tfrac{4}{10},\ \tfrac{11}{52},\ \tfrac{12}{13},\ \tfrac{3}{2},\ 1\tfrac{1}{2}$$

The correct answers are:

$$\tfrac{4}{10} = 0.4$$

$$\tfrac{11}{52} = 0.21$$

$$\tfrac{12}{13} = 0.92$$

$$\tfrac{3}{2} = 1.5$$

$$1\tfrac{1}{2} = 1.5$$

Observe that in the last two answers the procedure for converting the fraction to a decimal remains the same. These numbers are unique in that they are mixed numbers. The number $\frac{3}{2}$ was specifically selected to show that $\frac{3}{2}$ is the same as $1\frac{1}{2}$ which is the same as 1.5, and although a mixed number may appear, simply follow whichever arithmetic process is easier for you.

As a final refresher on decimals, let's discuss the identification of *place values*. Each position following the decimal point to the right is associated with a named place value.

XX.XXXX
whole number . parts of the whole number
whole numbers = one, two, tens, twenties, etc.
parts of the whole number = tenths, hundredths, thousandths, ten thousandths

1.1 is one and one-tenth
1.01 is one and one-hundredth
1.001 is one and one-thousandth
1.0001 is one and one-ten thousandths

Decimals

The fractional part is named by the last number beyond the decimal point. For example, 1.1 is one and one-tenth, 1.11 is one and eleven-hundredths (*not* one and eleven-tenths).

A zero as the last digit has no value significance. The number 1.10 is still one and one-tenth. However, 1.01 is one and one-hundredth.

Try reading this one: 10.1234. You should have read it as ten and one thousand two hundred and thirty-four ten-thousandths.

Practice Problems

1. A physician wants 10 capsules of a specially formulated drug. Each capsule is to contain 0.375 Gm. of the active ingredient. How many grams must be weighed out to prepare the physician's prescription?
2. The physician has ordered a patient to take a medication for 3 days. For the first 2 days the patient is to take $1\frac{1}{2}$ Gm. doses 3 times a day. For the last day the patient is to take only one dose that contains half the amount of the drug. How much drug will you need to prepare the order?
3. In problem 2 the prescription permits refills. You find that you have 19.9 Gm. of the drug in the bottle. How many times will you be able to refill this prescription with the amount of drug you have available?
4. How many grams are in the following doses? (Name the numbers.)
   (a) 0.025 Gm.
   (b) 2.74 Gm.
   (c) 10.001 Gm.
   (d) 1.1000 Gm.
   (e) 110.011 Gm.
5. Convert the following numbers to decimals (if a fraction) or to fractions (if a decimal):
   (a) $\frac{1}{10}=$
   (b) $0.125=$
   (c) $\frac{3}{4}=$
   (d) $0.11=$
   (e) $\frac{23}{4}=$

Answers

1. 0.375 Gm. of drug × 10 capsules prescribed = 3.750 Gm. total drug needed for 10 capsules
   (*Note:* The zero on the end of the decimal has no value. You would weigh out 3.75 Gm. of the drug.)
2. Three days = total.
   For each of the first two days:
   1.5 Gm. three times a day = 4.5 Gm. per day.
   For the first two days this will add up to 9.0 Gm.
   For the last day:
   One dose of half the amount is equal to 0.75 Gm.
   Total amount of drug needed = 9.75 Gm.
   (9.0 Gm. for the first two days + 0.75 Gm. for the last day.)
3. With 19.9 Gm. of drug on hand, you will be able to refill the prescription only one time (19.9 Gm./9.75 Gm. = 2.04 or enough drug for the original prescription plus one refill).

4. (a) 0.025 Gm. = twenty-five thousandths of a gram
   (b) 2.74 Gm. = two and seventy-four hundredths grams
   (c) 10.001 Gm. = ten and one-thousandth grams
   (d) 1.1000 Gm. = one and one-tenth grams
   (e) 110.011 Gm. = one hundred ten and eleven-thousandths grams
5. (a) $\frac{1}{10} = 0.1$
   (b) $0.125 = 125/1000$, which can be reduced to $\frac{1}{8}$
   (c) $\frac{3}{4} = 0.75$
   (d) $0.11 = \frac{11}{100}$
   (e) $\frac{23}{4} = 5.75$

PERCENTAGE

The next order of review is a mathematical expression which is very important to pharmacy practice. You often see drug products prepared in specific strengths expressed as a percentage. For instance, hydrocortisone ointment, lotions, and sprays come in strengths of 0.5% and 1%, phenylephrine nose drops are available in strengths of $\frac{1}{4}$%, $\frac{1}{2}$%, and 1%. Profits/loss, pricing, and many management applications are also expressed in terms of percentage.

Percentage is a method of expressing fractional parts. In pharmacy the use of percent is very common and useful. The basis of percent is that the *whole* is divided into 100 parts (percent is a Latin derivative meaning "by the hundred"). For instance, you know that one dollar is made of 100 individual pennies or cents. If you measure one cent as a part of the dollar, the result is 1 percent, or 1%. Similarly, if you take 50 cents of this dollar and express it as a percentage of the dollar, the result is 50%.

Logic may lead you to believe that the maximum which can be achieved is 100%, or the "whole thing." But you can exceed 100%. A five dollar bill, for example, is simply 5 times the one dollar bill, or 500%.

You may find percentages in excess of 100% when you evaluate profits or customer traffic. Pharmaceutical preparations, however, *do not* exceed a 100% concentration. A saturated solution of potassium iodide (KI) contains 1 gram (Gm.) of KI in each milliliter (ml.) of solution. This solution has a 100% concentration.

The values of percentages can also be less than 1%. It is very common to see drug preparations in concentrations of $\frac{1}{8}$%, $\frac{1}{4}$%, 0.5%, and so on. This should not be confusing as long as you adhere strictly to the basic mathematical operations using percentages.

What should you know to feel comfortable with percentages? There are three elements to percentage:

1. the resulting percent
2. the parts involved
3. the "whole" with which you are dealing

Percentage

In the application of percentages, you may be asked to find:

1. the *percent*, which is the part divided by the whole,
2. the *part*, which is the percent times the whole, or
3. the *whole*, which is the part divided by the percent.

Although the percent notation is commonly used to describe the parts of the whole or drug product concentration, it is necessary to convert this percent notation to a workable form, the decimal. This is easily accomplished by simply following the rule: *To change a percent to a decimal, move the decimal point two places to the left and drop the percent symbol.* For example, to change 21% to a decimal, move the decimal point two places to the left (21.0% becomes 0.21) and drop the % sign, resulting in a decimal 0.21 ($\frac{21}{100}$ is the fractional form). Observe that this system is based on 100.

The decimal fraction is the usable form for accomplishing the necessary mathematical operations you will encounter. Practice using decimal fractions until you feel comfortable with the operations. These calculations become critical in preparing intravenous formulations, among other pharmacy preparations.

Moving the decimal point two places to the left also works with numbers greater than 100%. Try the number 218%. What decimal would you use in working out a drug compounding problem? If you said 2.18, you are correct. The number 2.18 says:

1. 2.18 is 2.18 times greater than the "whole." If a manager says that the prescriptions in his department have increased by 218%, he is indicating an increase in prescription volume of 2.18 prescriptions for every prescription his department did previously.
2. 2.18 is the same as $2\frac{18}{100}$ or $\frac{218}{100}$
3. 2.18 is the decimal notation for 218%

Change the following percents to decimal fractions:

$$5\%, \tfrac{1}{2}\%, 32\%, 176\%, 4.87\%$$

Your decimal fractions should be:

$$0.05, 0.005, 0.32, 1.76, 0.0487$$

There are three basic types of percentage problems you will encounter. Follow the steps as they appear in each example.

A. *Find Percent:* What percent of 8 is 3?

Given: 8 = the whole, 3 = the part
Find: the percent
Operation: part/whole
$\frac{3}{8}$ = 0.375 (decimal fraction)
Convert the decimal fraction to a percent.

$0.375 \times 100 = \%$ (multiplying by 100 is the same as moving the decimal point two places to the right)

Answer: 37.5%

Rule. To change a number from a decimal to a percent, move the decimal point two places to the right and add the % symbol.

B. *Find the Part:* What number is 16% of 62?

Given: 16% = the percent, 62 = the whole
Find: the part
Operation: percent × whole

You cannot work with 16%. Therefore, you must convert 16% to a decimal fraction. Your decimal fraction is 0.16. $0.16 \times 62 = 9.92$, or 9.92 is the part of 62 that represents 16%.

C. *Find the Whole:* 60 is 4% of what number?

Given: 60 = the part, 4% = the percent
Find: the whole
Operation: part/percent

$\frac{60}{4\%} = 60/0.04 = 1500.0$, or 60 represents 4% of 1500

Did you notice the logic used to solve these examples? Working out word problems is often made easier by listing three major elements:

1. the information given,
2. what you are asked to find, and
3. the operation used to solve the problem.

Therefore, using scratch paper, restate the problem in a way you understand. Write the heading *Given* and list the information given, write the heading *Find* and state what you are seeking, and finally, solve the problem step-by-step with the information you have (including information found elsewhere such as conversions used in weights and measures).

Practice Problems

1. The owner of the pharmacy has purchased a quantity of vitamins for $108.00. The quantity consists of 2 cases with 24 bottles of vitamins in each.
    (a) If he sells each bottle for $2.95, what percent profit will the owner be making?

Percentage

(b) What percent of the bottles must be sold for the owner to break even (that is, make an amount of money equal to his investment of $108.00)?

(c) What price should each bottle sell for in order to realize a 50% profit on the owner's investment?

The following practice problems use percentages as they apply to pharmaceutical preparations.

2. The hospital in which you are working makes a number of its bulk products in the pharmacy. You are assigned to the pharmacy manufacturing room on the day the Minor Surgery Department needs more of its disinfecting solution. You review the pharmacy's compounding manual and find the following formula for bronchofibroscopic disinfecting solution (minor surgery): *instrument to goes thru lungs to check for cancer etc*

betadine — povidone-iodine solution 50%
70% ethyl alcohol 25%
distilled water 25%

Prepare a total volume of 4000 ml. How much of each ingredient will you need?

3. A special order is written by a physician in the Radiology Department. The order requires the pharmacy to prepare a Hypaque Solution in a 3.33% concentration. The pharmacy has bottles already prepared with 8 grams of Hypaque powder in each bottle. How much diluent must be added to the powder to prepare the prescribed preparation?

4. You receive a call from a physician who is concerned about the availability of calcium in a calcium preparation he or she is prescribing for a patient. You review the label on a bottle of calcium glucobionate and determine that there is 9.5% available calcium in 1200 milligrams (mg.) of calcium glucobionate. How many milligrams of calcium do you tell the physician are available?

5. The chief pharmacist has assigned you the special task of identifying the major causes of improperly completed prescriptions. You have identified the following problems as major reasons for improperly completed prescriptions:

(a) no refill instructions
(b) incomplete patient name
(c) missing addresses on prescriptions for controlled drug substances (including narcotics)
(d) out-of-date prescriptions
(e) inappropriate drug strengths
(f) illegible physician signature

After reviewing and tallying the prescriptions for a five-day period, you have gathered the following information:

Total number of prescriptions received: 637
Total number of prescriptions for controlled drugs and narcotics: 197 (this number is included in the 637 total count)
The number of prescriptions with problems contained in the major categories:
(a) no refill instructions: 142
(b) incomplete patient name: 299
(c) missing addresses on controlled prescriptions: 11

(d) out-of-date prescriptions: 7
(e) inappropriate strengths: 14
(f) illegible physician signature: 473

The chief pharmacist wants you to report to him the percent of prescriptions showing each problem. He will then take the necessary actions to correct the problems based on the degree of abuse. The results you present to the chief become very important. What does your report look like?

Answers

1. (a) Given: purchase price = $108.00
    quantity = 2 cases with 24 bottles per case
    (total of 48 bottles)
    selling price = $2.95
   Find: percent profit (the profit is the amount of money made in excess of the purchase price)
   Operations: $2.95 (selling price per bottle) × 48 (number of bottles)

   $141.60 (gross sales)
   −$108.00 (cost of merchandise)
   $33.60 (profit)

   $33.60/$108.00 = 31.1% profit made by the owner on his investment of $108.00.

   (b) Given: $2.95 = selling price per bottle
    $108.00 = owner's investment in 48 bottles
   Find: the number of bottles which must be sold to break even
   Operations: $108.00/$2.95 = 36.6 or 37 bottles (rounded off)

   To answer the question of what percent of the merchandise must be sold to break even, consider the number of bottles sold to break even as a percent of the total number of bottles purchased by the owner.

   $\frac{37}{48}$ = 0.77 or 77% of the merchandise must be sold before the owner starts to make a profit.

   (c) Given: $108.00 = purchase price of merchandise
    48 = number of bottles purchased
   Find: the selling price for each bottle of vitamins to result in a 50% profit to the owner.
   Operations: 50% of $108.00 = 0.50 × $108.00 = $54.00

   $108.00 owner's investment
   $54.00   50% profit
   $162.00 total sales required to give the owner a 50% profit on his investment

   Now, to determine the sales price for each bottle of vitamins:

   $162.00/48 = $3.38 selling price per bottle

   In other words, selling all 48 bottles at $3.38 each will give the owner a 50% profit ($54.00) on his investment of $108.00.

2. Given: total volume required is 4000 ml.
    % of each ingredient in formula
   Find: amount of each ingredient in the final product
   Operations: % × whole
   povidone-iodine solution: 50% × 4000 ml. = 0.50 × 4000 ml. = 2000 ml.

Percentage

70% ethyl alcohol: 25% × 4000 ml. = 0.25 × 4000 ml. = 1000 ml.
distilled water: 25% × 4000 ml. = 0.25 × 4000 ml. = 1000 ml.

Note: If you add up the amount of each ingredient in the problem, the result is a total of 4000 ml., the required amount to be prepared.

3. Given: Hypaque powder = 8 grams
required concentration = 3.33%
Find: volume of diluent required to make the preparation
Operations: part/percent

$$8/3.33\% = 8/0.0333 = 240 \text{ milliliters of diluent}$$

In other words, by adding 240 ml. of a diluent to the 8 grams of Hypaque, you will have a final solution containing a 3.33% concentration of Hypaque. Check your answer: $\frac{8}{240} = 0.0333$ or 3.33%.

4. Given: 1200 mg. of calcium glucobionate
9.5% available calcium
Find: amount of calcium available in the formulation
Operations: % × whole

$$9.5\% \times 1200 \text{ mg.} = 0.095 \times 1200 = 114 \text{ mg.}$$

You are able to inform the physician that there are 114 mg. of calcium available in every 1200 mg. of calcium glucobionate.

5. Given: 637 total prescriptions
197 controlled drug and narcotic prescriptions

Problem Category	Number of Problems
a	142
b	299
c	11
d	7
e	14
f	473

Find: percent each problem represents of all the problems
Operations: part/whole

(a) $\frac{142}{637} = 0.2229 = 22.29\%$ or 22.3%

(b) $\frac{299}{637} = 0.4693 = 46.93\%$ or 46.9%

(c) The total number of prescriptions in this problem category is only the number of controlled drug and narcotic prescriptions. Therefore, your whole number becomes 197 and you determine the percentage based on these specific prescriptions.

$$\frac{11}{197} = 0.0558 = 5.58\% \text{ or } 5.6\%$$

(d) $\frac{7}{637} = 0.0109 = 1.09\%$ or 1.1%

(e) $\frac{14}{637} = 0.0219 = 2.19\%$ or 2.2%

(f) $\frac{473}{637} = 0.7425 = 74.25\%$ or 74.2%

You have now provided the chief pharmacist with a substantial report. He will be able to establish a corrective action plan based on priorities set by these percentages.

RATIO AND PROPORTION

You have completed some very important basic mathematical tool reviews. You should feel comfortable with the concepts behind decimals and percentages and the way to use them properly. You have built the foundation for a commonly used mathematical operation in pharmacy called *ratio and proportion*.

By definition, a ratio is an expression of the relative value of one number to another. For example, the number $\frac{1}{2}$ shows the relationship between the numbers 1 and 2. The quantity 1 is half of the quantity 2.

Whole numbers also show a relationship between quantities. Take the number 2. Written as a ratio, "2" is expressed as $\frac{2}{1}$ or $2:1$ (*Note*: ratios may be written as fractions, or with a colon, :). The relationship in this instance is that the quantity "2" is twice as great as the quantity "1."

Two equal ratios form a proportion. Therefore, it is necessary to have four numbers to complete a proportion. Practically, a proportion may be defined as an extension of a ratio. Take the ratio $1:2$ or $\frac{1}{2}$. You know that $\frac{1}{2}$ is equal to $\frac{2}{4}, \frac{3}{6}, \frac{4}{8}$, and so on. Each of these ratios is equal to any other listed—$2:4::4:8$, $2:4::3:6$, $1:2::12:24$. When one ratio is set equal to another, this forms a proportion. For instance, $\frac{2}{4} = \frac{4}{8}$ is a proportion which shows that the relationship of each number in each ratio is the same. In the first ratio, $\frac{2}{4}$, 2 parts are half of the 4 parts. The same is true with the second ratio, in which 4 parts are half of the 8 parts. The ratios are equal even though the numbers are different. This proportion may also be written as $2:4::4:8$ (the colon means "is to"; the double colon means "as"). This equation is spoken as "2 is to 4 as 4 is to 8." The numbers 4 and 4 are called the means and the numbers 2 and 8 are referred to as the extremes.

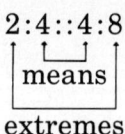

extremes

You will see the importance of applying your knowledge of proportions when you prepare different quantities of a drug from a given compounding order. You may need to determine new prices or amounts from given prices and amounts. Other applications are available also.

There are rules which are true for all proportions:

1. The product of the means equals the product of the extremes. Using the example of $2:4::4:8$, the product of the means or $4 \times 4 = 16$ and the product of the extremes or $2 \times 8 = 16$ are equal.
2. The product of the means divided by one extreme equals the other extreme. The product of the means or $4 \times 4 = 16$ divided by one of the extremes, 8, equals the other extreme, 2 (that is, $\frac{16}{8} = 2$).
3. The product of the extremes divided by one mean gives the other mean. The test of this rule will be left up to you to verify using our example.

Ratio and Proportion

In order to see how these rules apply, consider the following situation. A patron hands you a prescription for 100 tablets of pseudoephedrine 60 mg. (a nasal decongestant). You inform the patron that the prescription will cost her $16.00 for 100 tablets. The patron decides that she would prefer to try some of the medicine before purchasing the entire prescription. She asks for only 25 tablets. What do you charge for the 25 tablets?

You may reason that $16.00 for 100 tablets is equal to $0.16 per tablet ($16.00/100 tablets = the cost per tablet). Therefore, 25 tablets should logically cost $4.00 (25 tablets × $0.16 per tablet).

Using this example to illustrate the use of ratio and proportion may appear extreme for such a simple problem. However, a working skill of proportions will enable you to tackle and solve any problem with any degree of difficulty. Using the method of proportion, you can state the given information:

Given: 100 tablets = $16.00
Find: the charge for 25 tablets
Operations: set up a proportion

tablets/tablets as dollars/dollars
100:25::$16.00:? (? = unknown)

Referring to rule two, the product of the means divided by one extreme equals the other extreme.

25 × 16.00 divided by 100 = $4.00

Hint: Keep similar labels together. In this case you can associate tablets "is to" tablets as dollars "is to" dollars.

$4.00 for 25 tablets is the same as $16.00 for 100 tablets. The price for each tablet remains the same, but because the total quantity changed, there was a *proportional* change in the charge to the patron. Also, by keeping like labels together, you knew that solving for the unknown in this case was solving for dollars.

See if the other rules of proportion apply to this example. There are no gray areas in mathematics. Familiarize yourself with ratio and proportion. You will encounter the need for its use in solving pharmacy compounding problems, intravenous mixtures, pricing, and other non-pharmacy needs.

Complete the practice problems before continuing with the chapter on weights and measures.

Practice Problems

1. The nurse in the Newborn Intensive Care Unit (NICU) of the hospital calls the pharmacy with a request to determine how many milliliters (ml.) of calcium gluconate injection will provide 150 mg. of calcium. The vial of calcium gluconate states 9.3 mg. of calcium is contained in each milliliter. How many milliliters must the nurse administer to the infant patient to provide 150 mg. of calcium?

2. Referring to the first problem, if each calcium gluconate vial contains 10 ml., how many vials will be needed to provide the required amount of drug?

3. Again referring to the first problem, a medical student calls the pharmacy to find out how many milliequivalents (mEq.) of calcium are contained in the 150 mg. of calcium. After checking the appropriate sources (in this instance the label on the vial contains the mEq. content), you determine that 9.3 mg. of calcium equals 0.465 mEq. How many mEq. of calcium equals 150 mg. of calcium?

4. You are preparing bottles in the intravenous (IV) pharmacy when you receive an order for a change in flow rate (the rate at which the contents of an IV has been determined to flow into the patient) from 40 ml. per hour to 50 ml. per hour. Liter (1000 ml.) bottles are prepared for a 24-hour period. You have already prepared one bottle for the patient. Will the bottle be enough? If not, how many more will be required for the 24-hour period?

5. The owner of the pharmacy in which you are working has just purchased a "deal" on tubes of allergy cream. The deal consists of a gross (12 dozen or 144 individual pieces) of tubes of allergy cream. The owner of the pharmacy normally stocks 12 tubes of the cream and allots a foot and one-half of shelf space for them. The owner does not want to spare more than 24 inches of shelf space for the "deal." He wants you to figure out the number of tubes needed to stock the increased shelf space allotment. Also, if he sells 18 tubes of cream per week, how many weeks will the "deal" last?

Answers

1. 16.1 ml.
2. 1.61 vials. The pharmacy will send two vials of 10 ml.-size calcium gluconate to the NICU. The nurse will withdraw 16.1 ml. of calcium gluconate which will provide the required 150 mg. of calcium.
3. 7.5 mEq.
4. No. We know that 960 ml. of a 1000 ml. (one liter) bottle is used over a 24-hour period. Proceed to the next step and determine whether increasing the flow rate by 10 ml. per hour requires the preparation of additional bottles. Yes, one more bottle will be necessary although only a portion (200 ml.) will be used.
5. 16 tubes. An additional 4 tubes will be needed. *Hint:* Convert the measure to like labels. You cannot work with feet and inches. Change the labels to either feet or inches. This "deal" will last 8 weeks.

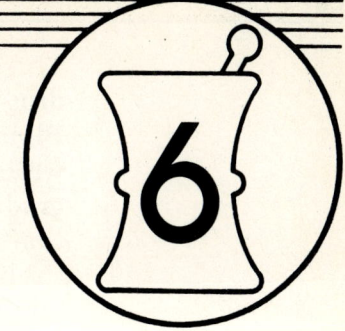

Pharmacy Computations

SYSTEMS OF MEASURE

Now that you have completed a review of the fundamental arithmetic operations important to pharmacy, you can proceed with the science of weights and measures known as *metrology* (from the Greek *metrologia*, meaning "theory of ratios"). The essence of pharmacy historically surrounded the accurate measurement of herbs and other medicinal ingredients used in preparing potions, salves, elixirs, and so on. Today, even though most drugs are premade, one of the fundamental activities of pharmacy remains the measurement of drug quantities for compounding medications. A knowledge of weights and measures is needed to properly adjust existing drug dosage strengths when necessary. The science dealing with medication dosages is called *posology*, from the Greek word *posos*, meaning "how much."

There are a number of measurement systems which have been used for pharmacy calculations. These include the apothecaries' system, metric system, Troy weight, avoirdupois, and even household measurements. Each system of measurement has established standards of weight and volume (except for avoirdupois, which measures weight only). However, since pharmacy deals with the measurement of minute quantities, only two systems could adequately be used to measure these small amounts. The systems are the apothecaries' system and the metric system. These two systems became the accepted measurements for drugs.

The metric system is currently the primary measurement used by drug companies and those involved in pharmacy practice. Dr. A. S. Blumgarten, author of *Textbook of Materia Medica and Therapeutics*, wrote, "In this country, the apothecaries' system is still used, but it is gradually being superseded by the metric system. It is simply a question of time when the apothecaries' system will be abandoned entirely." For this reason, pharmacy technicians should be aware and familiar with the apothecaries' system until such time that the system no longer exists for pharmacy.

In addition to the metric system and apothecaries' system, this chapter will look briefly at two other measures seen in pharmacy practice. The avoirdupois (pronounced avoe-du-pwah) and household measures are occasionally used in compounding and dosage directions on prescriptions, respectively. However, the extent of their value and use is so limited that it is important to remember only a few necessary measurements and their conversions to other systems.

The acceptance of the avoirdupois pound was the result of relations between France and England. The King of England adopted the avoirdupois pound, which is equivalent to sixteen ounces. The importance of the sixteen-ounce avoirdupois pound to pharmacy is only that it should not be confused with the twelve-ounce apothecary pound.

Historically, avoirdupois measure was used for bulk weights of raw drug products. Apothecary measure was used for much smaller drug quantities used in the actual compounding of specific medications.

Household measure is used primarily by patients who take medicine at home. Since they are not familiar with grams, milliliters, and fluid measures (such as fluid drams and fluid ounces), it becomes the pharmacist or pharmacy technician's responsibility to assure the person that he or she is taking the correct dosage. Therefore, it is necessary to know the equivalents among the various systems of measurement. The pharmacy technician will then be able to convert the dosage from "pharmacy language" to everyday household language which readily enables a person to take medication with a teaspoon, tablespoon, or dropper.

Tables 6-1 and 6-2 show the most common equivalents you will encounter.

TABLE 6-1

Common Pharmacy Conversions

Household	Apothecaries'	Metric
1 drop	1 minim	0.06 ml.
1 teaspoonful	1 fluid dram	4–5 ml.
1 tablespoonful	4 fluid drams	15 ml.
2 tablespoonsful	1 fluid ounce	30 ml.
1 glassful	8 fluid ounces	240 ml.

TABLE 6-2

Common Pharmacy Equivalents

Avoirdupois
437.5 gr. (gr. = grains) = 1 oz. (oz. = ounce)
7000 gr. = 16 oz. = 1 lb. (lb. = pound)

Apothecary
480 gr. = 1 ʒ (ʒ = ounce)
12 ʒ = 5760 gr. = 1 lb.

POINTS TO REMEMBER

1. A standard teaspoonful has been established to contain approximately 5 ml.
2. 60 gtt. (gtt. = drops) = 1 teaspoonful (also written 1 ʒ)
3. 3 teaspoonsful = 1 tablespoonful (also written ʒss, ss = $\frac{1}{2}$)
4. 1 teaspoonful = approximately 5 Gm. (Gm. = grams)
5. 1 teaspoonful = approximately 60 gr.

THE APOTHECARIES' SYSTEM

The standard unit of measure for weight (solid substances) in the apothecaries' system is the *grain* (abbreviated gr.). Fluids (liquid volumes) in the apothecaries' system are measured by the unit called the *minim* (abbreviated ℞.). You may see a number of different symbols used in apothecaries' measurement. Table 6-3 summarizes the most commonly encountered symbols and their meanings.

Occasionally a physician will write prescriptions using apothecaries' measure. However, this system has gradually been replaced by the metric system.

TABLE 6-3

Common Pharmacy Symbols

Symbol	Meaning
℞.	minim
ʒ	dram or drachm (pronounced dram)
fʒ	fluid dram, fluid drachm
ʒ	ounce
fʒ	fluid ounce
O or pt.	pint
qt.	quart
C or gal.	gallon
gr.	grain
℈	scruple
lb.	pound

Table 6-4 summarizes units used in the apothecaries' system.

TABLE 6-4

Common Apothecary Conversions

Capacity (fluid measure usually refers to liquids)	
60 minims	= 1 fluid dram
8 f℥	= 1 fluid ounce
16 f℥	= 1 pint
2 pints	= 1 quart
4 quarts	= 1 gallon

Weight (solids)	
60 gr.	= 1 dram (℈)
480 gr.	= 8 ℈ = 1 ounce (℥)

Note: The ℈ symbol and the ℥ symbol are used in both the dry and liquid apothecaries' measure. The letter f preceding the symbol denotes fluid for the liquid measure (f℥ or f℈).

THE METRIC SYSTEM

After the French Revolution, at the end of the eighteenth century, France adopted the metric system of measurement. In 1837, the French made the metric system a law and everybody in France was obliged to use this system. The United States Congress, in 1866, made the metric system legal in this country, even though the system was not commonly used here. Then, in 1890, the United States Pharmacopeia (USP) adopted metric measure. This action by the USP was especially important because the USP is the legally recognized compendium of standards for drugs.

The advantages of the metric system are that it is simple, brief, adaptable, and universal. There are metric measures for length, area, volume, weight, temperature, and even money. Pharmacy, however, is concerned mainly with weights and volumes of drugs.

The metric system is a decimal system which can be divided into any parts which are a multiple of 10 (10, 100, 1000, etc.). Greek and Latin prefixes are used to show what multiple is used. For instance, *milli* is a Latin prefix meaning one-thousandth ($\frac{1}{1000}$). Joining the prefix *milli* to the word *liter* (a measure of liquid volume) forms the word *milliliter* (abbreviated ml. or mL.), which means one-thousandth of a liter.

The standard unit of metric measure for capacity or volume is the *liter*. The *gram* is the standard unit of metric measure for weight. You have already seen how the Latin prefix *milli* was used to denote a portion of the unit measure, the *liter*. The other prefix commonly used is *centi*. This Latin prefix defines a unit measure to be one-hundredth ($\frac{1}{100}$) of the unit. Finally, an infrequently used Latin prefix is *deci*, which means one-tenth of the unit.

The most commonly used Greek prefix is *kilo*, which denotes "one thousand times" the unit. You will often see measures in kilograms, which equal 1000 times the grams (for example, 2 kilograms = 2000 grams). Drug manufacturers determine drug dosages using body weight measured in kilograms. For example, a 165-pound person weighs 75 Kg. (Kg. or kg. = kilogram). The kilogram label is often referred to as "kilos." A drug monograph (the profile of a drug which lists dosages, administration schedules, side effects, and much more) lists the amount of drug to be given based on the patient's weight in kilograms.

At one time I would have disregarded the unit of measure for length—the meter. However, over the last few years, developments have been made in dosage forms which are measured in linear measure. Two examples are a nitroglycerine ointment (abbreviated NTG or TNG ointment) and a nitroglycerine patch. You may encounter prescriptions for NTG ointment with a dosage measured in inches. Nitroglycerine patches are measured in square centimeters (cm.^{2}).

Although a patient may be directed to apply the nitro (jargon for nitroglycerine) ointment in inch measures, a resident doctor in a hospital may exercise his or her newly acquired metric expertise. The nitro patches, however, are actually measured in square centimeter areas—5 cm.^{2} (cm.^{2} = square centimeters), 10 cm.^{2}, 20 cm.^{2}, and so forth.

The following units, once memorized, will enable you to solve nearly all of those rarely occurring problems involving metric linear measure:

2.54 cm. (cm. = centimeter) = 1 inch
1 cm. = 0.01 M. (M. = meter)
1 mm. (mm. = millimeter) = 0.001 M.
meter = metric unit for linear measure
1 Km. (Km. = kilometer) = 1000 M.

There are two metric measures which predominantly apply to pharmacy. As a pharmacy technician, your primary use of metric measure will be for both the volume or cubic measure (for liquids) and weight measure (for solids) of drugs and medicinal ingredients used in compounding special prescription orders.

In the metric system, the unit of volume or capacity is the *liter* (abbreviated L. or l.). Large-volume solutions are referred to by their liter size. You may hear a nurse say she needs twenty K in a liter of D 5 W. What the nurse is saying is that she needs one liter of 5% of dextrose (a sugar) in water (D5W) with 20 milliequivalents of potassium (K) incorporated into the liter.

Liter-size intravenous preparations (IVs) are prepared by major pharmaceutical companies such as Travenol, McGaw, and Abbott Laboratories. Many different fluids are purchased in liter sizes. Such preparations include 5% dextrose in water (D5W), normal saline (NS), half-normal saline ($\frac{1}{2}$ NS), and 5% dextrose in normal saline (D5NS), and are among a vast variety of liters available from companies.

Other pharmacy activities involving metric volumetric calculations use fractional parts of the liter. These fractional parts are usually expressed in milliliters (ml.) or cubic centimeters (cc.). *The milliliter and cubic centimeter are equivalent.* In your practice of pharmacy, these designations are interchangeable. You will often see liter or milliliter measure. It is, therefore, very important for you to remember that:

$$1 \text{ liter} = 1000 \text{ milliliters}$$
$$1 \text{ milliliter} = 0.001 \text{ liter}$$

For example, 0.5 L. = 500 ml. or 500 cc.

The metric unit of weight is the *gram* (Gm., gm., or G.). The kilogram (1000 grams), originally used as the unit of weight, was too large to meet the practical needs of pharmacy. The gram has been standardized as the weight of 1 milliliter of distilled water at 4 degrees Celsius (centigrade). It is important that you remember:

$$1 \text{ gram} = 1000 \text{ milligrams}$$
$$1 \text{ milligram} = 0.001 \text{ gram}$$

The gram and the milligram are the most frequently used designations for weight measure in pharmacy practice. Note that the weight 0.250 Gm. may be read as "point two hundred and fifty grams" or 250 milligrams (1 gram = 1000 milligrams, 0.250 gm. × 1000 mg. per gram = 250 mg.).

Occasionally you will encounter a drug measured in micrograms (μg. or mcg.). Remember that:

$$1 \text{ Gm.} = 1{,}000{,}000 \text{ mcg.}$$
$$1000 \text{ mg.} = 1{,}000{,}000 \text{ mcg.}$$
$$1 \text{ mg.} = 1000 \text{ mcg.}$$
$$1 \text{ mcg.} = 0.001 \text{ mg.}$$

Thyroid agents such as levothyroxine and liothyronine are measured in both milligrams and micrograms. You will commonly see levothyroxine labels listing strengths of 25 mcg. (0.025 mg.), 50 mcg. (0.050 mg.), 100 mcg. (0.1 mg.), 125 mcg. (0.125 mg.), and so on, through 300 mcg. (0.3 mg.).

Microgram measure is also used in defining how a drug distributes itself in the body after it is absorbed. The distribution is measured in mcg./ml. (micrograms per milliliter). Traditional pharmacy drug references such as the *Physicians' Desk Reference* (PDR), *Drug Information* (a publication of the American Society of Hospital Pharmacists), and others contain information about these concentrations. The Minimum Inhibitory Concentration (MIC) of an antibiotic (the least amount of an antibiotic needed to inhibit the growth of a bacteria) is also measured in mcg. per ml.

You will frequently encounter Physician's Orders and prescriptions for special medications or dosage forms which require a conversion within the same system (for example, convert 0.350 Gm. to 350 mg.—the quantities are both metric, but for convenience you may find using milligrams preferable) or from one system to another (for example, convert 170 pounds to 77 kilograms because most drug dosage requirements are determined by body weight measured in kilograms). The translation of quantities from one system to another or within a system is called a *conversion*. Most physicians are not familiar with the various systems which exist and, therefore, write orders in a way which may appear to be jumbled quantities.

The pharmacy technician can easily adjust the Physician's Order and process it by knowing a few key conversions. We have already discussed the most common conversions within the metric system (liter/milliliters and gram/milligrams/micrograms). There are convenient equivalents which help you go from one system to another. These should be memorized. All pharmacy computations should be done in one system. The equivalents shown in Table 6-5 are used to bridge different measurement systems.

TABLE 6-5

Common Conversions

Linear Measure

1 meter (M.) = 39.37 inches
1 inch = 2.54 centimeters (cm.)
1 cm. = 0.39 inch

Fluid Measure

1 ml. = 16.23 minims (practical usage—rounded to 16 ℳ.)
1 fʒ = 29.57 ml. (practical usage—rounded to 30 ml.)
1 pt. = 473 ml. (practical usage—rounded to 480 ml.)

Weight Measure

1 Gm. = 15.432 gr. (practical usage—rounded to 15 gr.)
1 Kg. = 2.2 lbs.
1 gr. = 0.065 Gm. or 65 mg.
1 oz. (avoirdupois) = 28.35 Gm. (practical usage—rounded to 30 Gm.)
1 ʒ (apothecary) = 31.1 Gm. (practical usage—rounded to 30 Gm.)
1 lb. = 454 Gm.
1 oz. = 437.5 gr. (avoirdupois)
1 ʒ = 480 gr. (apothecary)

Liquid drug preparations, creams, and ointments are expressed as percentage concentrations. This simply means that a certain quantity of the drug or drugs is contained in the final quantity of the product. For instance, a 1% hydrocortisone cream contains 1 gram of the hydrocortisone drug in 100 grams of the final product (the drug plus the cream). A 5% sodium chloride (salt) solution contains 5 grams of sodium chloride in 100 milliliters of the final product (drug and distilled water). We already learned from our review of percents that 1 gram in

100 grams or 1/100 is equal to 0.01 or 1%. Similarly, 5 grams in 100 milliliters is equal to 5/100 or 0.05 or 5%.

In pharmacy, there are three ways of preparing a product which result in a percentage concentration. One method uses weight to weight (w/w) measurement. You can derive w/w percentage by dissolving a given quantity of ingredient (called the solute) in a liquid (called the solvent) measured in grams. W/w is also used in making creams and ointments with specific quantities of active ingredients. Percentage concentrations indicate the amount of active ingredient found in 100 grams of the solvent or cream. However, not every solution, cream, or ointment is 100 grams. As we learned, percentages can be established using any quantities. Consider the previous hydrocortisone (abbreviated HC) 1% cream example. Use 1 gram of HC and mix it thoroughly in 99 grams of cream. The result is a final preparation of 1 gram HC per 100 grams of total product. Note that any part of the HC 1% cream final product contains 1% HC. If you use 10 grams of a 100 gram jar, the 10 gram amount is a 1% HC preparation and the remaining 90 grams in the jar is a 1% HC cream. However, you will not usually be asked to make preparations in quantities convenient to the percentage system based on 100. HC 1% is usually prepared in 30-gram sizes.

How do you determine the necessary quantities of each ingredient for a 1% HC preparation?

Remember, 1% is also written as 0.01, HC is part of the entire product, and the entire product is 30 grams. The equation becomes:

$$\frac{\text{HC quantity}}{30 \text{ grams}} = 0.01$$

Solution:

$$\text{HC quantity} = 30 \text{ grams} \times 0.01 = 0.3 \text{ grams}$$

You now know that you need 0.3 grams (or 300 mg.) of HC in 29.7 grams of cream to make 30 grams of HC 1% cream.

This simple example indicates the use of w/w in some product formulations. As a rule, however, w/w is uncommon for liquid product formulations.

Weight to volume, designated w/v, is the method commonly applied to solution percentage concentrations. As in the w/w methodology, the active ingredient or solute is measured in grams. A sufficient quantity or volume of solvent, measured in milliliters, is added to make the required solution. Observe that w/v is not applicable to creams and ointments.

Using our previous sodium chloride 5% example, theoretically 5 grams of sodium chloride is measured and placed in a beaker, cone graduate, or cylindrical graduate (laboratory pieces of equipment containing imprinted calibrated lines and used for measuring). Enough solvent (for example, distilled water) is added to the sodium chloride to bring the level of the solution up to 100 ml. The 5 grams are dissolved in 100 ml. of finished product making a 5% solution. The weight part of w/v is measured in grams and the volume part of w/v is measured in milliliters. Since not all solutions are premeasured as 100 ml., the quantity of solute used to prepare any volume is easily computed using the same steps discussed for the w/w method of percentage concentrations.

Most sodium chloride solutions are prepared in liter sizes. Since 1 liter is equal to 1000 ml., calculate the amount of sodium chloride which will be needed to make 1 L. of 5% sodium chloride (sodium chloride is abbreviated NaCl). Following the same steps under the w/w method, you get:

$$\frac{\text{sodium chloride quantity}}{1000 \text{ ml.}} = 0.05$$

Solution:

$$\text{amount of NaCl needed} = 0.05 \times 1000 \text{ ml.} = 50 \text{ grams}$$

Therefore, 50 grams of sodium chloride is placed in a graduate or beaker and solvent is added to the 1000 ml. level. You have prepared a 5% sodium chloride solution.

Finally, there is the volume to volume, v/v, method used to determine a percentage concentration for liquid solutes dissolved in liquid solvents. This method measures the milliliters of an active ingredient (liquids are usually measured in terms of volume) to be incorporated in a total volume of the solution measured in milliliters. The percentage concentration is based on the milliliters of solute per 100 ml. of finished product. The mathematical operations are the same as those in the two previous examples.

A physician writes an order for a 5% solution of wintergreen oil in isopropyl alcohol. How much wintergreen oil will be needed to prepare 4 fluid ounces of the preparation?

You know:

1. You want a 5% solution of wintergreen oil.
2. You want a final amount of 4 fluid ounces.
3. Four fluid ounces equals 120 ml.

You need to know how much wintergreen oil is required to make the product.

The solution is:

$$\frac{\text{amount of solute}}{\text{quantity of finished product}} = 5\% = 0.05$$

Substituting where appropriate, you have

$$\frac{x}{120 \text{ ml.}} = 0.05$$

$$x = 0.05 \times 120 \text{ ml.} = 6 \text{ ml. of wintergreen oil}$$

Proceed to place 6 ml. of wintergreen oil in a beaker or graduate and stir in isopropyl alcohol until 120 ml. is attained.

Regardless of how you solve any percentage concentration problem, you must remember to express the relationship between the solute and solvent in the appropriate denomination, as shown in Tables 6-6 and 6-7.

TABLE 6-6

Metric Concentration Relationships

Methodology	Solute	Solvent
w/w	grams	grams
w/v	grams	milliliters
v/v	milliliters	milliliters

TABLE 6-7

Apothecary Concentration Relationships

Methodology	Solute	Solvent
w/w	grains	grains
w/v	grains	minims
v/v	minims or f℥	minims or f℥

In this chapter we discussed conversions, or the translation of quantities into forms which are workable for pharmacy computations. We discussed the various types of percentage concentrations and how each applies to pharmacy preparations.

One final conversion is often used in pharmacy and should be known. This is the temperature conversion from Fahrenheit to Celsius and vice versa. Sometimes the need to do so arises in bulk product manufacturing. Occasionally a patient may ask about a body temperature stated in Celsius. The following simple formula can be used to convert temperature either way by merely inserting the correct temperature:

$$\left(\tfrac{9}{5} \times {}^\circ C\right) + 32 = {}^\circ F$$

Examine the following example using body temperature. You know that normal body temperature is 98.6 measured in degrees Fahrenheit (°F). How would it be written in degrees Celsius (°C) (which is usually the case in the hospital setting)?

$$\left(\tfrac{9}{5} \times {}^\circ C\right) + 32 = 98.6$$
$$\left(\tfrac{9}{5} \times {}^\circ C\right) = 98.6 - 32$$
$$\tfrac{9}{5} {}^\circ C = 66.6$$
$${}^\circ C = 66.6 \text{ divided by } \tfrac{9}{5}$$
$${}^\circ C = 37$$

Therefore, 37°C = 98.6 °F.

A doctor tells a patient that she is to call if her temperature goes above 38°C. The patient realizes later that her thermometer is calibrated in Fahrenheit. She asks you to convert the Celsius temperature to Fahrenheit. What is 38°C equivalent to in °F?

$$\left(\tfrac{9}{5} \times {}^\circ\text{C}\right) + 32 = {}^\circ\text{F}$$
$$\left(\tfrac{9}{5} \times 38\right) + 32 = {}^\circ\text{F}$$
$$68.4 + 32 = {}^\circ\text{F}$$
$$100.4 = {}^\circ\text{F}$$

Therefore, $38\,^\circ\text{C} = 100.4\,^\circ\text{F}$.

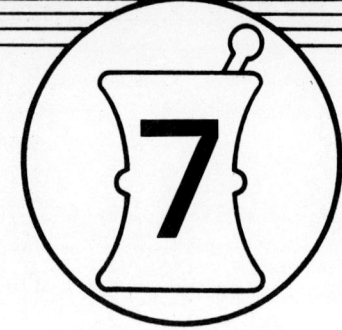

Drug Classes

This chapter deals with the primary focus of pharmacy—drugs. The Food and Drug Administration (FDA) estimates the number of drugs for which national codes exist to be around 35,000. How does anyone begin to learn about 35,000 drugs? Fortunately, only 200 drugs comprise approximately 75 percent of the drug market. Even learning about 200 drugs appears to be an enormous task.

We will direct our drug review to drug classes rather than individual drugs. Focusing on major drug classes will enable us to look at characteristics associated with each drug class and, therefore, there is a good possibility that each drug in the class will exhibit those characteristics. An additional advantage of studying drug classes is the large number of drugs with which you will become familiar.

The format of this chapter is designed to address each major class of drugs, with an introductory brief note followed by a list of categories and generic drugs representing each major class. Where subdivisions of a major class exist, generic drug representatives have been listed for each subdivision. The first class, for instance, defines analgesics as a major class. However, a number of subdivisions occur for analgesics and include salicylates (aspirin is the representative drug), para-aminophenol (acetaminophen is the representative drug), and narcotics (codeine is one of many representative examples listed). The narcotic analgesic subdivision has been further divided into specific groups based on the drug derivatives. Studying drugs to this extreme may not be practical or necessary for the purposes of this text. However, the information is available and provided for your review.

Drugs, as a rule, are not absolute by category. Many drugs exhibit crossover therapeutic activity. Nonsteroidal anti-inflammatory agents (NSAIA) may be classified as analgesics because they reduce pain responses. NSAIAs are also considered to be anti-inflammatory agents and antiarthritic agents.

There is a lack of absolute consistency in drug classification. Drugs may be classified according to the therapy they elicit (for example, pain-killing), the disorder for which they are intended (for example, antidiarrheal), the pharmacologic response (for example, antihistamine) or the anatomical/physiological effect they have (for example, anatomic: cardiovascular agents; physiological: diuretic).

The best way to facilitate learning the massive amounts of information about drugs is to review each class. Highlight important features associated with each group. Learn the names of the most commonly used drugs in each group. Interrelate information where possible and, above all, *keep current* by reading drug journals and other drug literature.

Following are thirty major drug classes. Trade names have not been included because it is common for drug patents to expire (patents are valid for seventeen years). Once a drug patent has expired, many drug manufacturers ("drug houses") may produce the generic form of the drug using their own coined names for the drug. The generic name, however, does not change.

Identifiers used in the following listings are as follows:

Major drug groupings (for example, antibactcrials) are identified by a capital letter.

Subdivisions within a major drug grouping (for example, cephalosporins) are identified by a number.

Generic drug representatives have no identifiers.

ANALGESIC

Analgesics are characteristically used to treat pain. Some analgesics are also able to reduce fever (antipyretic properties), reduce inflammation, and/or inhibit blood platelet aggregation. Some narcotic analgesics (for example, codeine) are used to suppress coughs.

Representative Categories and Drugs

A. Salicylates
   aspirin — Ecotrin
B. Para-aminophenol
   acetaminophen — Tylenol
C. Narcotic analgesics
   1. phenanthrene derivatives
      codeine   oxycodone
      hydrocodone   butorphanol
      hydromorphone   oxymorphone

ANALGESIC (Continued)

        levorphanol   nalbuphine
        morphine   pentazocine (not considered a narcotic)

2. phenylpiperidine derivatives
    alphaprodine
    anileridine
    fentanyl
    meperidine
    sufentanil
3. diphenylheptane derivatives
    methadone
    propoxyphene (not considered a narcotic)

Nonsteroidal anti-inflammatory agents (NSAIA) possess analgesic properties. As a class of drugs, they will be found under antiarthritic agents.

ANTIDIARRHEAL

Antidiarrheal drugs function to slow intestinal mobility and propulsion. The body interprets diarrhea as a positive response because it may be the only way of eliminating toxins. The problem with diarrhea, however, is the loss of excessive water and electrolytes, which can result in dehydration.

Representative Categories and Drugs
1. adsorbents
    kaolin and pectin
2. piperidine derivatives
    diphenoxylate
    loperamide
3. bacterial derivatives
    lactobacillus acidophilus
4. opiate derivative
    opium

ANTIHISTAMINE

Drugs of this class neutralize the effects of histamine (that is, edema, redness, and itching). These effects are allergic responses. The ethylenediamine group of antihistamines characteristically produce more adverse gastrointestinal (GI) upset than the other groups. Some antihistamines, especially the ethanolamine group, possess antiemetic properties. This same group also causes a high incidence of drowsiness while showing a low incidence of GI distress. The propylamine group causes less drowsiness and more central nervous stimulation than the other groups. Although phenothiazine drugs have antihistamine properties, they are used principally for their psychotherapeutic effects. In

ANTIHISTAMINE (Continued)

addition to antihistamine properties, drugs in this class are also used to treat motion sickness (for example, meclizine), anxiety and pain (for example, hydroxyzine), restlessness (for example, diphenhydramine, promethazine), pruritus (for example, chlorpheniramine), and nausea (for example, prochlorperazine).

Representative Categories and Drugs

1. ethylenediamine derivatives
    methapyrilene
    pyrilamine
    tripelennamine
2. ethanolamine derivatives
    carbinoxamine   diphenhydramine
    clemastine   doxylamine
    dimenhydrinate   phenyltoloxamine
3. propylamine derivatives
    brompheniramine   pheniramine
    chlorpheniramine   triprolidine
    dexbrompheniramine
4. phenothiazine derivatives
    methdilazine
    promethazine
    trimeprazine
5. piperazine derivatives
    buclizine   hydroxyzine
    cyclizine   meclizine
6. butyrophenone derivative
    terfenadine

ANTI-INFECTIVE

Anti-infective drugs include a large spectrum of agents used to support the body's defense mechanism or directly defend the body against bacterial, fungal, viral, and other biotic invasion. The terms antibiotic and antibacterial have been used interchangeably. Anti-infectives are comprised of specific classifications based on their primary chemical derivations, such as aminoglycosides, cephalosporins, beta-lactams, and more.

Representative Categories and Drugs

A. Antibacterial
   1. aminoglycosides
        gentamicin   tobramycin
        neomycin   kanamycin
        streptomycin   amikacin
   2. cephalosporins
        (Classification by "generation" represents similar activity against bacteria by each drug in the group.)

ANTI-INFECTIVE (Continued)

    (first generation)
      cefadroxil   cephalothin
      cefazolin   cephapirin
      cephalexin   cephradine
    (second generation)
      cefaclor   ceforanide
      cefamandole   cefoxitin
      cefonicid   cefuroxime
    (third generation)
      cefoperazone   ceftizoxime
      cefotaxime   ceftriaxone

3. beta-lactams
    moxalactam (chemically related to
      third-generation cephalosporins)
    ceftazidime (structurally related to
      beta-lactams, pharmacologic properties
      of third-generation cephalosporins)
    penicillins
      ampicillin   methicillin
      amoxicillin   nafcillin
      carbenicillin   oxacillin
      cloxacillin   penicillin
      dicloxacillin   ticarcillin
      hetacillin

4. tetracyclines
    demeclocycline   minocycline
    doxycycline   oxytetracycline
    methacycline   tetracycline

5. sulfonamides ("sulfas")
    sulfacytine   sulfasalazine
    sulfamethizole   sulfisoxazole
    sulfamethoxazole

6. sulfones
    dapsone
    sulfoxone

7. cephamycin
    cefoxitin (pharmacologic
      properties of second-
      generation cephalospo-
      rins)

8. urinary antiseptics
    methenamine   nitrofurantoin
    nalidixic acid   trimethoprim

9. miscellaneous
    (bacterial derivatives)
      bacitracin   polymixin B
      colistin   polymixin E

ANTI-INFECTIVE (Continued)

        chloramphenicol   "lincomycins"
        erythromycin   clindamycin
        novobiocin   lincomycin
        spectinomycin   folate-antagonist
        troleandomycin   trimethoprim
        vancomycin

B. Antiviral
   acyclovir
   amantadine
   vidarabine

C. Antifungal
   clotrimazole   griseofulvin
   ketaconazole   amphotericin B
   miconazole   nystatin
   butoconazole

D. Antituberculars
   aminosalicylic acid   capreomycin
   ethambutal   cycloserine
   pyrazinamide   rifampin
   ethionamide   streptomycin
   isoniazid

E. Antiprotozoans
   chloroquine   pyrimethamine
   iodoquinol   sulfadoxine/pyrimethamine
   hydroxychloroquine paromomycin
   metronidazole

F. Antiparasitics
   pyrantel   mebendazole
   pyrvinium   thiabendazole

ANTINEOPLASTIC

Chemotherapy is a treatment modality using chemical agents. These chemical agents produce a desired and anticipated therapeutic effect. The term has been associated with the treatment of cancer. The treatment of cancer is so complex that new terminology has been added steadily. Terms such as antimetabolite, cytotoxic, immunosuppressive, oncolytic, tumorcidal, and mutagenic are only a few representing the vast approaches which have been taken to treat cancer and the terminology which has resulted from new research. A popular basis for treatment is interference with the cancer cell's life cycle. Therefore, many chemotherapeutic agents exert their effects on the cancer cell's enzyme system used in proliferating cell growth through DNA synthesis.

ANTINEOPLASTIC (Continued)

Representative Categories and Drugs

A. Antimetabolites
   1. folic acid antagonists
      methotrexate
   2. purine antagonists
      azathioprine
      mercaptopurine
      thioguanine
   3. pyrimidine antagonists
      floxuridine
      fluorouracil
      cytarabine
   4. vinca alkaloids
      vinblastine
      vincristine
   5. urea derivative
      hydroxyurea

B. Alkylating agents
   1. nitrogen mustards
      chlorambucil   melphalan
      cyclophosphamide   uracil mustard
      mechlorethamine
   2. ethylenimines
      thiotepa
   3. alkylsulfonates
      busulfan
   4. triazenes
      dacarbazine
   5. nitrosoureas
      carmustine
      lomustine
   6. piperazines
      pipobroman

C. Antineoplastic antibiotics
   dactinomycin   mitomycin
   daunorubicin   bleomycin
   doxorubicin   plicamycin

D. Hormones
   1. adrenals
      prednisone
      prednisolone
   2. androgens
      dromostanolone
      testolactone

Cardiovascular

ANTINEOPLASTIC (Continued)

    3. Leuteinizing Hormone-Releasing Factor (LHRF)
        leuprolide
    4. estrogens
        diethylstilbestrol (DES)
    5. progestogens (progestins)
        medroxyprogesterone
        hydroxyprogesterone
        megestrol

E. Enzymes
    asparaginase

F. Miscellaneous
    mitotane
    procarbazine
    tamoxifen

ANTIULCER

The drug therapy used for ulcers attempts to promote healing of ulcerations by neutralizing acids, reducing the production of acids, or enhancing a barrier protection against the effects of acids.

Representative Categories and Drugs

1. anticholinergics

amsotropine	methantheline
clindinium	methscopolamine
glycopyrrolate	oxyphencyclimine
hexocyclium	oxyphenonium
isopropamide	propantheline
mepenzolate	tridihexethyl

2. H_2-receptor antagonists
    cimetidine *Tagamet*
    ranitidine *Zantac*

3. disaccharide
    sucralfate

CARDIOVASCULAR

The use of cardiovascular agents depends on the proper diagnosis by a physician. These agents vary widely, from influencing the contractility of heart muscle to affecting the consistency of blood.

Representative Categories and Drugs

A. Inotropics (affect heart muscle contraction)
    1. cardiac glycosides
        digoxin
        digitoxin
    2. beta-adrenergic agonists
        dobutamine
        isoproterenol

CARDIOVASCULAR (Continued)

   3. miscellaneous
      - dopamine
      - amrinone

B. Antiarrhythmics (stabilize the cardiac beat rhythm)
   1. nonspecific adrenergic blocker
      - bretyllium
   2. beta-adrenergic blocking agents
      - propranolol
      - nadolol
      - acebutolol
   3. alkaloid
      - quinidine
      - papavarine
   4. calcium channel blockers
      - diltiazem
      - nifedipine
      - verapamil
   5. amides/amines
      - lidocaine
      - procainamide
      - tocainide
      - disopyramide
      - flecainide
      - methoxamine
   6. sodium channel blockers
      - disopyramide

C. Antianginals (promote adequate blood and oxygen supply to the heart)
   1. calcium channel blockers
      (see drugs under *Antiarrhythmics*)
   2. nitrates
      - erythrityl tetranitrate
      - isosorbide dinitrate
      - nitroglycerin
      - pentaerythritol tetranitrate
   3. beta-adrenergic blockers
      (see drugs under *Antiarrhythmics*)
   4. miscellaneous
      - dipyridamole (non-nitrate)

D. Antihypertensives (reduce elevated blood pressure)
   1. alpha-adrenoceptor agonist
      - guanfacine
      - clonidine
      - guanabenz

E. Vasodilators (affect dilation of blood vessels)
   (see nitrate/nitrite drugs, non-nitrate, and alkaloid drugs under *Antianginals*)

F. Antilipemics (reduce the level of fatty substances in the blood)
   - cholestyramine
   - dextrothyroxine

CARDIOVASCULAR (Continued)

    clofibrate   gemfibrozil
    colestipol   probucol

DIURETIC

Diuretics are used to eliminate excessive fluid from the body tissues. These drugs are likely to be seen in the treatment of hypertension, edema, congestive heart failure, and glaucoma. Diuretics are categorized by structure (for example, thiazide diuretics) or action (for example, carbonic anhydrase inhibitors).

Representative Categories and Drugs

1. thiazide diuretics
   - chlorothiazide
   - hydrochlorothiazide
   - metolazone
   - methyclothiazide
   - trichlormethiazide
2. loop diuretics
   - ethacrynic acid
   - furosemide (Lasix)
   - bumetanide
   - chlorthalidone
3. osmotic diuretics
   - mannitol
   - urea
4. potassium-sparing diuretics
   - amiloride
   - spironolactone
   - triamterene
5. indolines
   - indapamide
6. carbonic anhydrase inhibitors
   - acetazolamide
   - dichlorphenamide
   - methazolamide
7. sulfonamide diuretics
   - acetazolamide
   - furosemide
   - indapamide

HORMONE

Hormones are very potent chemical substances. Only minute amounts of hormones are required to effect a response. Many hormones are available for many hormone-related disorders. Many hormone drugs exhibit variable mineralocorticoid and glucocorticoid properties.

Representative Categories and Drugs

A. Adrenocorticosteroids
   1. mineralocorticoids
      - desoxycorticosterone
      - fludrocortisone

HORMONE (Continued)

2. glucocorticoids
   - beclomethasone
   - betamethasone
   - cortisone
   - dexamethasone
   - flunisolide
   - hydrocortisone
   - meprednisone
   - methylprednisolone
   - paramethasone
   - prednisolone
   - prednisone
   - triamcinolone

(*Note*: fludrocortisone has properties associated with both mineralocorticoids and glucocorticoids. However, fludrocortisone is used primarily for its mineralocorticoid properties.)

B. Sex hormones
   1. androgens (male)
      - oxymetholone
      - methyltestosterone
      - fluoxymesterone
   2. estrogens (female)
      - ethinyl estradiol
      - diethylstibestrol
      - estradiol
      - quinestrol
      - chlorotrianisene
   3. progestins (female)
      - progesterone
      - medroxyprogesterone
      - norethindrone

C. Gonadotropins
   - chorionic gonadotropin
   - leuprolide
   - menotropin

D. Pituitary (human growth hormone)
   - somatropin
   - vasopressin

E. Thyroid
   - calcitonin
   - thyroid extract
   - levothyroxine
   - liotrix
   - liothyronine
   - thyroglobulin

F. Antidiabetic agents
   - insulin

   (*drugs used to stimulate insulin production*)
   - acetohexamide
   - chlorpropamide
   - glipizide
   - glyburide
   - tolazamide
   - tolbutamide

LAXATIVE

Laxatives promote the evacuation of feces from the intestine. Drugs function in a variety of ways to evacuate feces. Drugs have been developed to create "bulk" in the intestine, soften the stools in the intes-

LAXATIVE (Continued)

tine, lubricate the intestine, or stimulate the peristaltic action of the intestinal tract.

Representative Categories and Drugs
1. bulk laxatives
    methylcellulose
    carboxymethylcellulose
    psyllium
2. stool softeners
    docusate
3. saline laxatives
    magnesium citrate
    magnesium sulfate
    sodium phosphate
4. hyperosmotic laxatives
    sorbitol
    lactulose
5. intestinal stimulants
    bisacodyl   phenolphthalein
    cascara sagrada   danthron
6. intestinal lubricants
    mineral oil

PSYCHOTHERAPEUTIC

These agents are used for a variety of conditions associated with the mind and brain. They affect the central nervous system (CNS). Drugs are available for depression, anxiety, hyperactivity, and a number of other mental disorders.

Representative Categories and Drugs

A. Antidepressants
  1. monoamine oxidase (MAO) inhibitors
      isocarboxazid
      phenelzine
      tranylcypromine
  2. tricyclic compounds
      imipramine   nortriptyline
      desipramine   protriptyline
      trimipramine   doxepin
      amitriptyline   amoxapine
  3. tetracyclic compounds
      maprotiline
      trazodone
  4. phenothiazines
      promethazine   thiethylperazine
      ethopropazine   trifluoperazine

PSYCHOTHERAPEUTIC (Continued)

    propriomazine   thioridazine
    chlorpromazine   mesoridazine
    methotrimeprazine   methdilazine
    promazine   chlorprothixene
    triflupromazine   thiothixene
    trimeprazine   droperidol
    acetophenazine   haloperidol
    fluphenazine   loxapine
    perphenazine   molindone
    prochlorperazine

B. Stimulants

    amphetamine   mazindol
    benzphetamine   methamphetamine
    dextroamphetamine   methylphenidate
    diethylpropion   pemoline
    fenfluramine   caffeine
    phendimetrazine   doxapram
    phenmetrazine   nikethamide
    phentermine

C. Sedatives/hypnotics/anxiolytics

1. barbiturates

    amobarbital   pentobarbital
    aprobarbital   phenobarbital
    butabarbital   secobarbital
    mephobarbital   talbutal
    methohexital

2. benzodiazepines

    alprazolam   lorazepam
    chlordiazepoxide   oxazepam
    clorazepate   prazepam
    diazepam   temazepam
    flurazepam   triazolam
    halazepam

3. miscellaneous

    chloral hydrate   methyprylon
    ethchlorvynol   hydroxyzine
    chlormezanone   methotrimeprazine
    ethinamate   promethazine
    meprobamate   propiomazine
    glutethimide

HYPOTENSIVE

The term "hypotensive agent" denotes the desired results of this class. Drugs used to treat hypertension control high blood pressure. Physicians approach the treatment of high blood pressure (HBP) in steps:

HYPOTENSIVE (Continued)

1. oral diuretic (usually a thiazide)
2. sympathetic depressant (for example, beta-blocker, methyldopa, or reserpine)
3. vasodilator
4. another sympathetic depressant (for example, clonidine or guanethidine)

Representative Categories and Drugs
1. beta-adrenergic blockers
   - atenolol
   - acebutolol
   - metaprolol
   - timolol
   - pindolol
2. Angiotensin-Converting Enzyme (ACE)
   - captopril
   - enalapril
3. alpha- and beta-adrenergic blocker
   - labetalol
4. thiazide derivative
   - diazoxide
5. postganglionic adrenergic blockers
   - guanadrel
   - guanethidine
6. alpha-adrenergic blockers
   - prazosin
7. monoamine oxidase (MAO) inhibitors
   - pargyline
8. natural derivatives
   - reserpine
   - deserpidine
9. miscellaneous
   - clonidine
   - minoxidil
   - guanabenz
   - nitroprusside
   - hydralazine
   - mecamylamine
   - methyldopa
   - trimethaphan

ANTI-INFLAMMATORY

Anti-inflammatory agents are used for a variety of purposes. They may be used by those suffering from menstrual cramps, inflamed joints, or muscular spasms. Nonsteroidal anti-inflammatory agents (NSAIA) constitute the primary group within this class, because side effects are tolerable or preventable and the benefits are great.

Representative Categories and Drugs
A. Steroidal
   (see *Hormone* class for drug representatives)
   adrenocorticosteroids

ANTI-INFLAMMATORY (Continued)

    B. Nonsteroidal
       1. salicylates
          aspirin
          diflunisal
       2. nonsalicylates

fenoprofen	mefenamic acid
ibuprofen	phenylbutazone
naproxen	piroxicam
indomethacin	sulindac
meclofenamate	tolmetin

ANTIGOUT

Gout is a metabolic disorder characterized by inflammation of the joints resulting from uric acid crystals. It follows, therefore, that research would focus on a mechanism to eliminate excessive uric acid from the blood. That path was followed, resulting in a small, but reliable group of drugs.

Representative Categories and Drugs

1. xanthines
    allopurinol
2. natural derivatives
    colchicine
3. sulfonamide derivatives
    probenecid
4. miscellaneous
    sulfinpyrazone

MUSCLE RELAXANT

Muscle relaxants are prime examples of drugs that experience crossover in identification. There are skeletal muscle relaxants, smooth muscle relaxants, GI tract relaxants, genitourinary (GU) tract relaxants, and respiratory muscle relaxants. Muscle relaxants, for example, may be found under drugs for the gastrointestinal tract or respiratory tract. However, the various classifiers categorize muscle relaxants as agents that ultimately relax skeletal muscle (for example, voluntary muscle) or smooth muscle (for example, involuntary muscle).

Representative Categories and Drugs

1. skeletal muscle relaxants

baclofen	cyclobenzaprine
carisoprodol	diazepam
chlorphenesin	metaxalone
chlorzoxazone	methocarbamol

MUSCLE RELAXANT (Continued)

    2. smooth muscle relaxants
      (*GI tract*)
        loperamide
        diphenoxylate
      (*GU tract*)
        flavoxate
        oxybutynin
      (*Respiratory*)
        theophylline
    3. miscellaneous
      succinylcholine
      pancuronium

BRONCHODILATOR

Most bronchodilator drugs are sympathomimetics. These drugs function at the nerve sites, which stimulate the relaxation of smooth muscle. By relaxing these muscles, the passageways in the lung are permitted to expand, thereby enabling a greater air flow. Older compounds stimulated the heart muscle while effecting response in the bronchial smooth muscle. Newer drugs have been developed to reduce or avoid the unwanted effects on the heart muscle.

Representative Categories and Drugs

    1. sympathomimetic drugs (adrenergics)
        albuterol   isoproterenol
        bitolterol   metaproterenol
        ephedrine   terbutaline
        isoetharine
    2. nonsympathomimetics (xanthines)
        theophylline
        aminophylline

SUPPLEMENT

Supplements may be classified as nutritional (vitamins), electrolytic (potassium, sodium, calcium, chloride, etc.), and mineral, which in the general sense may refer to electrolytes. In a stricter sense, however, minerals may be construed as those elements which do not possess an electrical charge. Calcium as an electrolyte has an electrical charge of two (Ca^{++}), but as a mineral is referred to as elemental calcium (no electrical charge).

Representative Categories and Drugs

    1. vitamins
        single vitamin preparations   multiple vitamins with
        multiple vitamin prepara-   minerals
          tions   prenatal vitamins

SUPPLEMENT (Continued)

      pediatric vitamins with fluoride
      pediatric vitamins
      geriatric vitamins
      therapeutic vitamins

2. electrolytes
   - phosphorus
   - phosphate
   - potassium
   - calcium
   - sodium
   - chloride
   - magnesium
   - acetate
   - lactate

3. minerals
   - zinc
   - iron
   - copper
   - iodine
   - calcium
   - magnesium
   - manganese

ANTICONVULSANT

Anticonvulsant drugs function by raising the threshold to stimuli which initiate seizures. The anticonvulsant drugs available are used in the treatment of epilepsy. It should be noted that seizures can occur as a result of conditions other than epilepsy (that is, drug-induced seizures, tumor, etc.)

Representative Categories and Drugs

1. barbiturate derivatives
   - phenobarbital
   - primidone
   - mephobarbital
   - metharbital

2. benzodiazepine derivatives
   - clonazepam
   - clorazepate
   - diazepam
   - lorazepam

3. hydantoins
   - phenytoin
   - mephenytoin
   - ethotoin
   - phenacemide

4. miscellaneous
   - trimethadione
   - paramethadione
   - ethosuximide
   - methsuximide
   - phensuximide
   - carbamazepine
   - valproic acid
   - divalproex

ANTIARTHRITIC

Drugs found within this class are used to treat disorders of a larger magnitude called *collagen diseases*. These diseases affect the joints, skin, and supporting tissue of various organs. Many of the drugs used for inflammation are found in this class.

ANTIARTHRITIC (Continued)

Representative Categories and Drugs

A. Steroids
   1. adrenocorticosteroids
      prednisone
      cortisone
      hydrocortisone

B. Nonsteroidal anti-inflammatory agents (NSAIA)
   1. salicylates
      aspirin
      diflunisal
      salsalate
   2. nonsalicylates
      fenoprofen   mefenamic acid
      ibuprofen   phenylbutazone
      naproxen   piroxicam
      indomethacin   sulindac
      meclofenamate   tolmetin

C. Gold derivatives
      auranofin
      aurothioglucose
      gold sodium thiomalate

D. Heavy-metal antagonists
      penicillamine

E. Immunosuppressants
      azathioprine

F. Antimalarial agents
      chloroquine
      hydroxychloroquine

OPHTHALMIC

Sometimes referred to as optic drugs, these agents are used primarily for inflammation, infection, glaucoma, anesthesia, and diagnostics. These drugs <u>should be sterile and free from particulate matter</u>. All products used for the eyes should be in solution. Some drugs are available for both the ear as a suspension and the eye as a solution. These drugs are not interchangeable.

Representative Categories and Drugs

A. Anti-inflammatory agents
   1. steroids
      dexamethasone   medrysone
      fluorometholone   prednisolone
      hydrocortisone

OPHTHALMIC (Continued)

      2. nonsteroids
         epinephrine   propylhexedrine
         naphazoline   tetrahydrozoline
         oxymetazoline   xylometazoline
         phenylephrine   zinc sulfate

  B. Anti-infective agents
     1. antibacterials
        bacitracin   polymixin B
        chloramphenicol   sulfacetamide
        erythromycin   tetracycline
        gentamicin   tobramycin
        neomycin
     2. antifungal
        natamycin
     3. antiviral
        idoxuridine
        trifluridine
        vidarabine

  C. Antiglaucoma
     1. carbonic-anhydrase inhibitors
        acetazolamide
        dichlorphenamide
        methazolamide
     2. miotics
        acetylcholine   isoflurophate
        carbachol   physostigmine
        demecarium   pilocarpine
        echothiophate

  D. Anesthetic agents
     tetracaine
     proparacaine

  E. Diagnostic agents
      demecarium bromide   tropicamide
      echothiophate iodide   homatropine
      fluorescein   phenylephrine
      isoflurophate   hydroxyamphetamine
      cyclopentolate

  F. Lubricants/artificial tears
     hydroxypropyl cellulose
     methylcellulose

  G. Miscellaneous agents
    timolol
    epinephrine
    glycerine

HYPOGLYCEMIC

Hypoglycemic agents are used to treat hyperglycemic (diabetic) conditions. In many diabetics, the insulin-producing portion of the pancreas does not function properly. Hypoglycemic agents stimulate these cells (beta cells) to produce adequate insulin needed for the metabolism of carbohydrates.

Representative Categories and Drugs

1. sulfonylureas
   - acetohexamide
   - chlorpropamide
   - glipizide
   - glyburide
   - tolazamide
   - tolbutamide
2. hormones
   - insulin

ANTINAUSEANT/ANTIEMETIC

Drugs in this class include those which are used for motion sickness and vertigo. There are numerous causes of vertigo, nausea, and vomiting. Pregnancy, toxins, microbial infections, and radiation are only a few of the causes. In each situation, the approach to treatment is symptomatic. The drugs used alleviate the symptoms and not the cause. The purpose for these drugs is to provide comfort for the patient until other treatment dealing with the cause takes effect, resulting in the elimination of nausea, vomiting, or vertigo.

Representative Categories and Drugs

A. Antihistamine derivatives
   - diphenhydramine
   - meclizine
   - cyclizine
   - dimenhydrinate
   - hydroxyzine
   - promethazine
   - trimethobenzamide

B. Antidopaminergic derivatives
   1. phenothiazines
      - chlorpromazine
      - promazine
      - triflupromazine
      - fluphenazine
      - perphenazine
      - prochlorperazine
      - thiethylperazine
   2. miscellaneous
      - haloperidol
      - metoclopramide

C. Marijuana derivatives
   - nabilone
   - dronabinol

BLOOD MODIFIER

Blood-modifying drugs represent a multitude of agents used for almost anything involving the blood. If the problem is anemia, there are iron preparations. If the blood is too thick, anticoagulants are available to remedy the situation. There is even a drug to treat calf muscle pain due to an inadequate blood supply.

Representative Categories and Drugs

A. Antianemic agents
   - iron preparations
   - cyanocobalamine
   - folic acid

B. Anticoagulant agents
   1. coumarin derivatives
      - dicumarol
      - phenprocoumon
      - warfarin
   2. miscellaneous
      - anisindione
      - heparin

C. Hemostatic agents
   - aminocaproic acid
   - antihemophilic factor
   - factor IX complex
   - thrombin

D. Hemorrheologic agent
   - pentoxifylline

E. Thrombolytic agents
   - streptokinase
   - urokinase

ANTISPASMODIC

Spasms are sudden, involuntary muscle contractions. The drugs in this group focus primarily on gastrointestinal spasms and urinary spasms. Muscle relaxants focus on spasms occurring in the skeletal muscles.

Representative Categories and Drugs

A. Gastrointestinal
   1. natural alkaloids
      - atropine
      - belladonna
      - hyoscyamine
   2. semisynthetic derivatives
      - homatropine
      - methscopolamine

ANTISPASMODIC (Continued)

3. synthetic
   - anisotropine
   - clidinium
   - glycopyrrolate
   - hexocyclium
   - isopropamide
   - mepenzolate
   - methantheline
   - oxyphenonium
   - propantheline
   - tridihexethyl dicyclomine
   - oxyphencyclimine

B. Urinary
   1. natural alkaloids
      - atropine
      - hyoscyamine
   2. synthetic compounds
      - flavoxate
      - oxybutinin

ANTIPARKINSON

Parkinson's Disease is characterized by a progressive central nervous system involvement. Shaking is perhaps the most characteristic symptom. The disease occurs in the middle-aged and elderly, and eventually may become incapacitating. Drug treatment provides only symptomatic relief.

Representative Categories and Drugs

1. anticholinergic agents
   - benztropine
   - biperiden
   - cycrimine
   - hyoscyamine
   - procyclidine
   - trihexyphenidyl
2. antihistamine agents
   - chlorphenoxamine
   - diphenhydramine
   - orphenadrine
3. phenothiazine derivative
   - ethopropazine
4. dopamine-releasing drug
   - amantadine
5. dopamine-elevating drugs
   - levodopa
   - levodopa/carbidopa

ANTITUSSIVE

Antitussive compounds are used to treat coughing. Coughing can be due to many factors, but the symptomatic treatment is the same. Most drugs are effective at the central nervous system site (that is, the

ANTITUSSIVE (Continued)

"cough center"). Some drugs may work at the site of irritation causing the cough.

Representative Categories and Drugs

A. Centrally-acting agents
   1. narcotic derivatives
      codeine
      hydrocodone
   2. non-narcotic derivatives
      dextromethorphan
      diphenhydramine
B. Peripherally-acting agents
      benzonatate (non-narcotic)
      noscapine (non-narcotic)

OTIC

Otic agents are drugs intended specifically for the ear. Preparations are available to treat inflammation, infection, pain, and accumulated cerumen (wax).

Representative Categories and Drugs

1. anti-inflammatory agents
hydrocortisone	prednisolone
dexamethasone	desonide
2. analgesic agents
   benzocaine
   pramoxine
   antipyrine
3. anti-infective agents
chloramphenicol	acetic acid
colistin	domiphen
neomycin	parachlormetaxylenol
polymixin B	
4. cerumenolytic
   triethanolamine polypeptide
   carbamide peroxide
5. decongestant
   phenylephrine

DERMATOLOGIC

Dermatology has one of the most elusive groups of diagnoses. However, there are many drugs available to combat the wide variety of disorders associated with the skin and hair.

DERMATOLOGIC (Continued)

Representative Categories and Drugs

A. Anti-inflammatory agents

fluocinonide	triamcinolone
fluocinolone	desoximetasone
amcinonide	desonide
dexamethasone	clocortolone
diflorasone	flurandrenolide
hydrocortisone	halcinonide
betamethasone	methylprednisolone

B. Antihistamine agents
- diphenhydramine
- chlorcyclizine
- tripelennamine

C. Anti-infective agents
1. antibacterial

clindamycin	polymixin B
tetracycline	bacitracin
chloramphenicol	mafenide
erythromycin	povidone-iodine
nitrofurazone	silver sulfadiazine
gentamicin	iodoquinol
neomycin	iodochlorhydroxyquin
gramicidin	

2. antifungal

nystatin	ciclopirox olamine
iodochlorhydroxyquin (clioquinol)	clotrimazole
	miconazole
iodoquinol	econazole
griseofulvin	thiosulfate
triacetin	tolfanate
amphotericin B	zinc undecylanate
haloprogin	

3. antiviral/antiherpes agents
    - acyclovir
4. scabicide agents
    - crotamiton
    - lindane
5. pediculicide agents
    - lindane
    - pyrethrins/piperonyl butoxide

D. Antiacne agents
- benzoyl peroxide
- isotretinoin
- sulfur

DERMATOLOGIC (Continued)

    E. Antiseborrhea agents
        chloroxine   salicyclic acid
        coal tar   selenium
        sulfur   zinc pyrithione

    F. Antipsoriasis agents
        coal tar
        anthralin

    G. Miscellaneous
       1. depigmenting agents
           monobenzone
           hydroquinone
       2. repigmenting agents
           methoxsalen
           trioxsalen
       3. keratolytic agent
           salicyclic acid
       4. sunscreen
           para-aminobenzoic acid (PABA)
       5. topical analgesic/anesthetic agents
           benzocaine   dibucaine
           pramoxine   dyclonine
       6. cell-stimulating agent
           tretinoin
       7. debridement agents
           collagenase   fibrinolysin/desoxyribonu-
           dextranomer   clease
           sutlains

VAGINAL

Most gynecologic disorders involve the vagina. Inflammation, discharge, and bleeding are a few common symptoms which require the physician to choose from an assortment of vaginal preparations. Perhaps the most common problem associated with the vagina is the fungal infection.

Representative Categories and Drugs

    1. antifungal agents
        clotrimazole
        nystatin
        miconazole
    2. antitrichomonal agent
        metronidazole
    3. antibacterial agents
        "sulfonamides"
        triple sulfa

VAGINAL (Continued)

4. hormone agents
   dienestrol
   estropipate
   conjugated estrogens

ANTIOBESITY

Obesity is characterized by the accumulation of excessive body fat. Obesity is not considered a disease in the sense of how we traditionally view diseases. The cause of obesity is the consumption of more calories than are expended. Therefore, drug therapy (anorectic drugs) attempts to convince the individual that he or she is not hungry and can consume less food.

Representative Categories and Drugs
1. amphetamine agents
   benzphetamine
   dextroamphetamine
   methamphetamine
2. nonamphetamine agents
   diethylpropion   phentermine
   fenfluramine   mazindol
   phendimetrazine   phenylpropanolamine
   phenmetrazine
3. satient agents
   cholecystokinin   guar gum
   carboxymethylcellulose vegetable bran

Intravenous Pharmacy

HISTORY OF INTRAVENOUS THERAPY

The earliest history of treating illness intravenously dates back to 1492. Historical writings indicate the use of blood transfusion from three boys to Pope Innocent VIII. In 1615, Andreas Libavius promoted the use of silver tubes to carry blood from one individual to another.

It was not until 1628, with the publication of William Harvey's theory of circulation, that great attention was given to scientific research on intravenous-type treatment. For instance, in 1654 Francesco Folli successfully accomplished the method of transfusion by using a combination of silver tube, bone cannula, and animal blood vessel. The first successful direct transfusion from animal to animal occurred in 1665 by the English physician Richard Lower.

Sir Christopher Wren introduced medications into animals intravenously for the first time in 1656. He used medicaments such as opium, ale, and wine. His experiments whetted the curiosity of other researchers, such as Robert Boyle and Timothy Clarke, who carried on the investigation of intravenous therapy.

A number of obstacles precluded intravenous treatments from achieving uninterrupted progress and successful accomplishments. These included the inability to isolate drug compounds, the lack of knowledge about ways to purify drugs, and the frequent infections associated with using veins as a route to administer drugs.

As a result of the work by Pasteur and Lister on sterilization and aseptic technique, medical literature began to note the importance of sterilization, and of the need to sterilize the tools of intravenous therapy (syringes, tubes, bottles) and the solutions. Filters appeared on the scene. New attempts were made at packaging drug solutions aseptically.

A French pharmacist, Stanislaus Limousin, developed the first container for storing sterile preparations. He called this glass container the "ampoule," which is still in use today.

Modern day intravenous drug therapy began during the early twentieth century. In 1910, Paul Ehrlich developed a drug for the treatment of syphilis. Arsphenamine, as it was called, was his 606th compound—also known as the magic bullet or "606." Intravenous treatment was on its way. The era of chemotherapy had begun. *The National Formulary* (the authoritative book of pharmacy) recognized the first injectable solutions and made them official in its 1926 edition.

Overview

Diseases have always existed. The vast armamentarium of treatments and drugs, however, have not. Ironically, as technology advances, so does the complexity of treatment for many diseases. I have heard the statement, *the more we learn, the less we know*. We really know a lot more than ever before. However, through learning we realize that there is so much more to learn, with a multitude of questions always arising and yet to be answered.

We would logically believe that the compounding of drugs ended with modern day manufactured dosages and mass-prepared drugs. In reality, the advancement of medicine has revitalized the need for compounding—this time, in the form of parenteral therapy. Intravenous therapy, as part of the total concept of parenteral therapy, has been dramatic in both its acceptance by the medical practitioners and as a standard treatment modality. See Figure 8-1.

ADVANTAGES AND DISADVANTAGES

ADVANTAGES OF PARENTERAL ROUTES

1. Immediate drug effect—it is especially significant in conditions such as respiratory airway disease, cardiac arrest, and shock.
2. Avoids digestive secretions—some drugs (for examples, insulin and some antibiotics) are inactivated by enzymes in the gastrointestinal tract.
3. Method of treating unreactive patients—it is often necessary to use a parenteral form of drug in patients who are uncooperative, unconscious, or unable to swallow.
4. Assure compliance in some ambulatory patients—all drugs require compliance with a dosage schedule for successful treatments. Some drugs (for example, antibiotics) require absolute compliance for a successful outcome. In the case of some ambulatory patients, a practitioner may select a long-acting (sustained release) parenteral form of a drug to assure the correct amount of drug is used over a specific period of time. Injectable intramus-

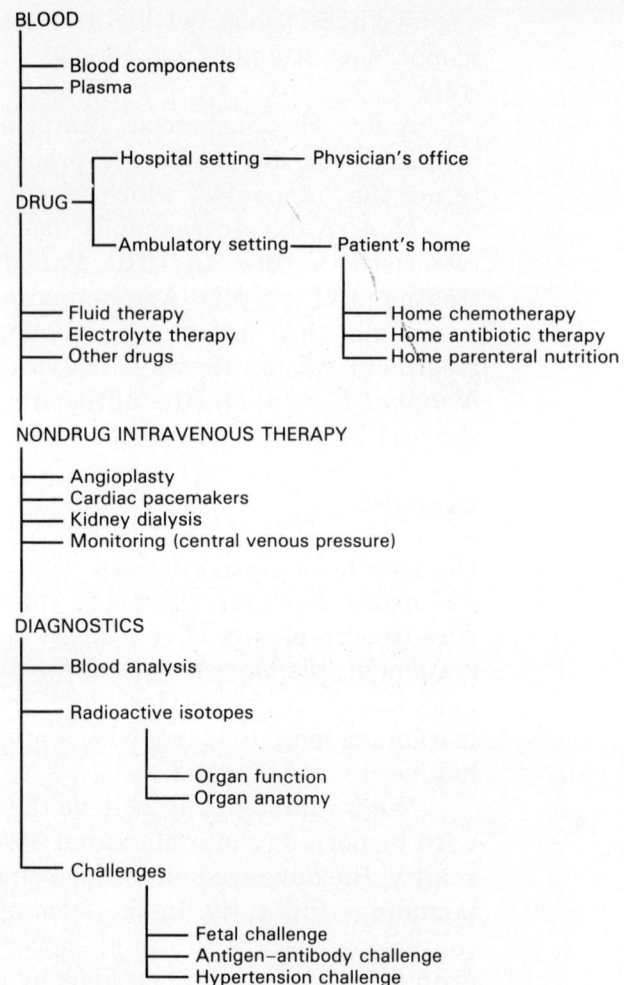

Figure 8-1 The spectrum of parenteral therapy.

cular penicillin suspensions are prime examples of long-acting parenteral formulations.

5. Localize treatment areas—there are times when a patient requires only a specific area to be treated. For example, a cortisone injection into a joint to relieve inflammation, an epinephrine injection into cardiac muscle to treat a cardiac arrest, or local nerve blocks with anesthetic drugs such as lidocaine.
6. Present as the sole treatment—intravenous therapy may be the only way to treat serious fluid and electrolyte imbalances, stubborn infections, or the only form in which some drugs are manufactured.
7. More predictable treatment—effective outcomes are more predictable as a result of a drug's rapid action. A practitioner has timely flexibility if a change of therapy is necessary.

DISADVANTAGES OF PARENTERAL THERAPY

1. Requires trained personnel to administer drug
2. Requires strict aseptic technique

3. Rapid effects may be irreversible
4. Usually more expensive than oral formulations
5. Less drug stability than oral formulations
6. Increased risk of infection, septicemia, clinically significant drug interactions, clotting mishaps, and breakdown of tissue (necrosis) surrounding the injection site
7. Requires patient hospital stay for most intravenous therapies

As a result of the greater risks associated with intravenous therapy, legal responsibilities mandate total competence. Increased reliance on pharmacy technicians for many facets of pharmacy, including intravenous admixtures, requires learning as much as possible and adhering to hospital protocol.

This chapter deals with a generalized academic exposure to parenteral therapy. Specific guidelines for preparing intravenous admixtures, the specific products purchased by hospitals, in-house protocols, and so on, will be determined by the facility at which you are gaining valuable practical experience while providing significant services. Intravenous therapy is a highly dynamic area of medicine. It is continuously subject to change due to the many ongoing improvements in medical practice, drugs, and equipment.

ANATOMY AND PHYSIOLOGY OF INTRAVENOUS THERAPY

At this time you may find it helpful to review portions of Chapter 4. Since this chapter deals specifically with intravenous therapy, you need only review the integumentary system and the cardiovascular/circulatory system.

The parts of the human anatomy which impact most significantly on intravenous drug administration are the skin, muscle, and circulatory system. Figure 8-2 shows the configuration of the layers comprising the skin portion of the integumentary system. The various routes of drug injection administration are also noted for each layer.

Figure 8-3 indicates additional layers below the subcutaneous tissue layer and the identification of specific routes of drug administration. Note the location of veins surrounded by muscle. Some drugs are manufactured specifically for intramuscular (IM) use. Practitioners administering parenteral medications must exercise extreme caution and avoid injecting IM preparations into a vein.

The circulatory system includes blood, lymph fluid, and the vessels through which they pass. The lymphatic system functions to return tissue fluid (called lymph fluid upon return to the lymphatic vessels) to the blood. Currently, there are no drugs which are indicated for specific injection directly into the lymph vessels. Blood serves to dilute parenteral drugs and transport these drugs throughout the body. All drugs administered by commonly used injection sites will eventually find their way to the blood stream where they will be carried along to exert their effects at the appropriate sites. Table 8-1 summarizes

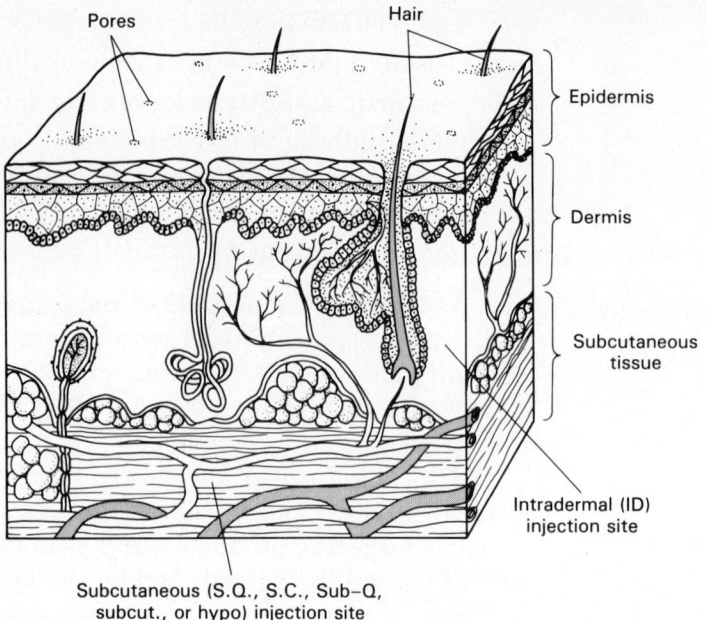

Figure 8-2 Cross section of cutaneous layers.

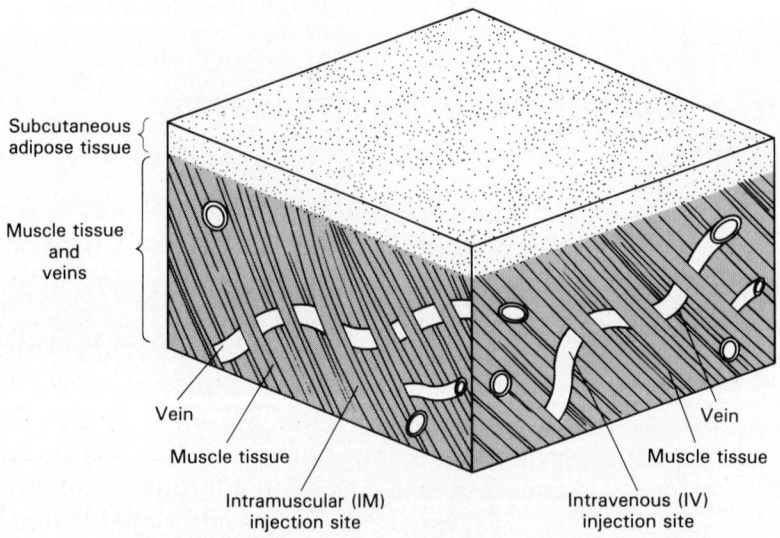

Figure 8-3 Cross section of subcutaneous layer and muscle tissue.

parenteral drug injection sites. Review Table 8-2 for a summary of the anatomy and physiology used in intravenous therapy.

An organism in perfect working order has proper balance, or *homeostasis*. This means that the body fluids contain all the essential elements in the correct proportions. Body fluids are comprised mostly of water and electrolytes ("lytes"), as follows:

ESSENTIAL VITAMINS

Water-soluble
    thiamine (B1)   biotin

riboflavin (B2)
niacin or nicotinic acid (B5)
pantothenic acid
pyridoxine (B6)
folic acid
cyanocobalamine (B12)
ascorbic acid (vitamin C)

Fat-soluble
vitamin A
vitamin D
vitamin E
vitamin K

TABLE 8-1

Parenteral Drug Routes

Route	Abbreviation	Notes
Intradermal	ID	Small drug volumes (0.1 ml.) are administered into the dermal layer of skin.
Subcutaneous, hypodermic	S.Q., S.C., Sub-Q, subcut., hypo	Small drug volumes are administered into the subcutaneous layer of the outer surface of the arm or thigh.
Intramuscular	IM	Up to 2 ml. volumes of drug may be administered into the muscle of the upper arm. Up to 5 ml. volumes may be administered into the muscle of the buttocks.
Intravenous	IV	Injection into the vein. Volume of drug is not a major factor. Drug effect, predictability, and dosage requirement impact on volume.
(Less frequently used routes)		
Intra-arterial		Into an artery ending at a specific site in a target organ
Intracardiac		Into the heart
Intra-articular		Into a joint
Intraspinal		Into the spine
Peridural		Into the area around the spine
Intrathecal		Into the spinal fluid
Intrasynovial		Into the fluid surrounding a joint
Hypodermoclysis		Large volume of fluid into the subcutaneous tissue layer

TABLE 8-2

Anatomy and Physiology Involved in Intravenous Therapy

Structure	Function
Skin	Protects, maintains moisture, responds to stimuli, eliminates waste, regulates body temperature
Blood vessels	Carry blood throughout the body; arteries carry blood away from the heart, while veins carry blood toward (into) the heart
Blood	Supplies body cells with oxygen, nutrients, and chemicals which regulate body functions; carries waste products to organs which eliminate wastes
Cells	Basic building blocks for each type of body organ

TRACE ELEMENTS

zinc (Zn)
copper (Cu)
chromium (Cr)
manganese (Mn)
selenium (Se)
molybdenum (Mo)
cobalt (Co)
iodine (I)

The Food and Drug Administration (FDA) acceptable standards for multiple trace element solution additives are:

zinc	4 mg.
copper	0.5 mg.
chromium	10 mcg.
manganese	0.15 mg.

The ideal total body water content is approximately 70 percent of body weight. The body fluids can be further divided into the fluid inside the cells (intracellular), at 50 percent, and outside the cells (extracellular), amounting to 20 percent. Extracellular fluid is comprised of fluid located in the spaces between the tissues (interstitial) and intravascular fluid in the blood (plasma).

The normal body fluid distribution may be upset by infection, age, environmental trauma, or genetic-related disorders. A fluid/electrolyte imbalance can cause a number of abnormal body states.

COMMON STATES OF BODY FLUID/ELECTROLYTE IMBALANCE

sodium excess (hypernatremia)
sodium deficit (hyponatremia)
water loss (dehydration)
acid-base imbalance (acidosis/alkalosis)
potassium deficit (hypokalemia)
potassium excess (hyperkalemia)
magnesium deficit (hypomagnesemia)
magnesium excess (hypermagnesemia)

The physician is trained to evaluate imbalances in a patient. He or she must consider many factors before selecting the appropriate therapeutic defense action (for example, intravenous antibiotic, chemotherapy), regulating action (for example, antiulcer, anti-inflammatory, fluid/electrolyte therapy), or nutritional support (for example, total parenteral nutrition or partial parenteral nutrition). The physician, with the aid of pharmacy technology, will select a treatment to correct profound alterations in anatomical or physiological derangements in fluid balance. See Figure 8-4.

TOOLS OF THE TRADE

Modern technology has provided a variety of therapeutic tools in the form of fluids, drugs, and equipment. Inasmuch as the objective of this

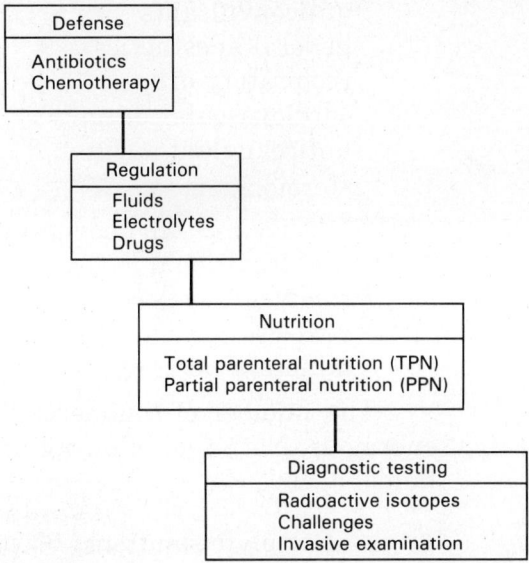

Figure 8-4 Intravenous therapy selection.

text is to develop an understanding of the parenteral components and their functions, we will review fluid therapy generically.

Since the seventeenth century, the parenteral/intravenous modality evolved from blood transfusions, going through stages which included the instillation of drugs, diagnostic techniques, and intravenous feeding. Associated with this increasing and advancing spectrum of intravenous tools are improvements in technology—from the historical silver tubes to today's modern computerized volumetric intravenous pumps.

There are a multitude of solutions used for IV therapy which vary enormously in contents, volumes, and use. The basic large-volume fluids include solutions of dextrose, sodium chloride, electrolytes, fats, and amino acids. Small-volume drugs are also available commercially. They include vitamins, trace elements, and many drugs for different treatments. Many drugs must be added to large-volume solutions for dilution. The resulting product is known as an admixture. The drug added to the large-volume solution is called an additive or "ad."

Selection of Therapy

FLUIDS: Restore and maintain homeostatic body fluid balance.
Examples:
    Plasma expanders:
        dextran   plasma
        hetastarch   normal human serum
        lactated Ringer's injection   albumin

DRUGS: Restore regulatory processes, defend against invading pathogens, and relieve symptoms associated with disorders.
Examples:
    antimicrobial drugs   antihypertensive drugs
    analgesics   diuretics

anticonvulsants
general anesthetics
respiratory drugs
cardiovascular drugs
anticoagulant agents
steroid agents

thrombolytic drugs
hormones
antiulcer drugs
antineoplastic (oncolytic) drugs

NUTRIENTS: Sustain body processes while patient is unable to ingest and/or use traditional foods.

Examples:
dextrose
minerals/electrolytes
trace elements
amino acids

The number of commercially available intravenous solutions is enormous. Note the following sample of commonly used intravenous fluids.

Single electrolyte solutions:

- sodium chloride 0.45%, $\frac{1}{2}$NS, 0.5NS (*Note:* NS may appear as S) (also called half normal saline or hypotonic saline)
- sodium chloride 0.9%, NS (also called normal saline or physiological saline or isotonic saline)
- sodium chloride 3%
- sodium chloride 5%
  (*Note:* any sodium chloride (salt) concentration greater than normal saline solution is a *hypertonic* solution)
- sodium lactate
- sodium bicarbonate 5%

Dextrose solutions:

- dextrose 5% in water, D5W
- dextrose 10% in water, D10W
- dextrose 20% in water, D20W

Combination dextrose and electrolyte solutions:

- dextrose 2.5% and sodium chloride 0.45%, D2.5 $\frac{1}{2}$S
- dextrose 5% and sodium chloride 0.2%, D5 $\frac{1}{4}$S
- dextrose 5% and sodium chloride 0.45%, D5 $\frac{1}{2}$S, D5 0.5S
- dextrose 5% and sodium chloride 0.9%, D5S, D5NS
- dextrose 5% + potassium chloride (KCl) in a variety of concentrations
- dextrose 5% + $\frac{1}{2}$NS + KCl

Other preparations are commercially formulated to include other concentrations of dextrose, sodium chloride, and other electrolytes (for example, dextrose 5% in Ringer's solution or lactated Ringer's solution).

Multiple electrolyte solutions:

- lactated Ringer's solution (Hartmann's solution)
- Ringer's solution

Amino acid solutions:

- amino acid solutions
- amino acids + dextrose
- amino acids + dextrose + electrolytes

Fat emulsions for intravenous use:

- products are available in 10% and 20% concentrations

Other available fluids:

- invert sugar in water
- invert sugar and electrolytes
- fructose in water
- fructose and electrolytes
- dextran in dextrose solution
- dextran in sodium chloride solution
- sodium lactate $\frac{1}{6}$M (M = molar)
- sterile water for injection

See Appendix F for commonly used diluents.

Electrolyte preparations are also available in single small quantities. For example, you will usually find potassium chloride (KCl) in 10 ml. or 20 ml. vials containing 20, 30, or 40 mEq. These products must be diluted before use. They allow the physician greater flexibility in adjusting concentrations for specific electrolytes. See Figure 8-5 for commonly used electrolytes.

Nutritional Support

Nutrient solutions are used in patients who are unable to ingest, digest, or absorb nutrients from the gastrointestinal tract. Patients who have undergone surgery usually require a short-term intravenous feeding. In these cases the objective is to supply enough carbohydrates (approximately 150 grams/day) to prevent protein breakdown, maintain brain metabolic activities, and assure erythrocyte metabolism. Dextrose solutions in low concentrations of 5% or 10% with sodium chloride in concentrations of 0.25% or 0.45% (that is, D5 $\frac{1}{4}$S, D5 $\frac{1}{2}$S, D10 $\frac{1}{4}$S, or D10 $\frac{1}{2}$S) are the usual fluid selections. These solutions are infused through a peripheral vein.

Patients may require a modified parenteral feeding for a short time in order to sustain the body's metabolic functions. This modified nutritional support program is called *partial parenteral nutrition (PPN)*. A PPN therapy requires an amino acid solution (a nitrogen source) with a low dextrose concentration (up to 10%) optional. Some

Anions / Cations	HCO$_3$	Cl	PO$_4$	SO$_4$	gluconate	acetate	lactate
Na	NaHCO$_3$	NaCl				Na acetate	Na lactate
K		KCl	*				
Ca		CaCl			Ca gluconate		
Mg				MgSO$_4$			
NH$_4$		NH$_4$Cl					

*Commercial preparations of potassium phosphate injections contain a mixture of monobasic potassium phosphate (KH$_2$PO$_4$) and dibasic potassium phosphate (K$_2$HPO$_4$).

Figure 8-5 Commonly used electrolyte additives. These electrolyte preparations are available in small quantities and may be used in varying amounts, giving the physician greater flexibility in adjusting concentrations of commercially available preparations.

practitioners may prescribe a fat emulsion to be added to the PPN regimen. The PPN is infused through a peripheral vein.

PARTIAL PARENTERAL NUTRITIONAL REGIMENS

- amino acid (supplies nitrogen) and dextrose (supplies carbohydrate)
- amino acid, dextrose, and fat emulsion (supplies calories)
- amino acid solution alone

Long-term intravenous total nutritional support is indicated for patients with excessive protein deficits. *Parenteral hyperalimentation* or *total parenteral nutrition (TPN)* is a therapy which provides the patient with all the nutritional requirements to support the functions of life. TPN is comprised of amino acids and a high concentration dextrose as a fundamental solution, and is infused through a central venous route. The central venous route is necessary because the blood flow is greater, thereby diluting the concentrated TPN solution rapidly. The practitioner, after a thorough assessment of the patient and laboratory values, prescribes specific concentrations or quantities of electrolytes, vitamins, minerals and trace elements to be added to the TPN solution. See Figure 8-6.

Fat emulsions are also available and are used as a nonprotein source of calories in addition to the dextrose. Fat emulsions are given intravenously through a separate intravenous line.

Intravenous preparations present a part of pharmacy which is vast and constantly changing. The knowledge you acquire, the techniques

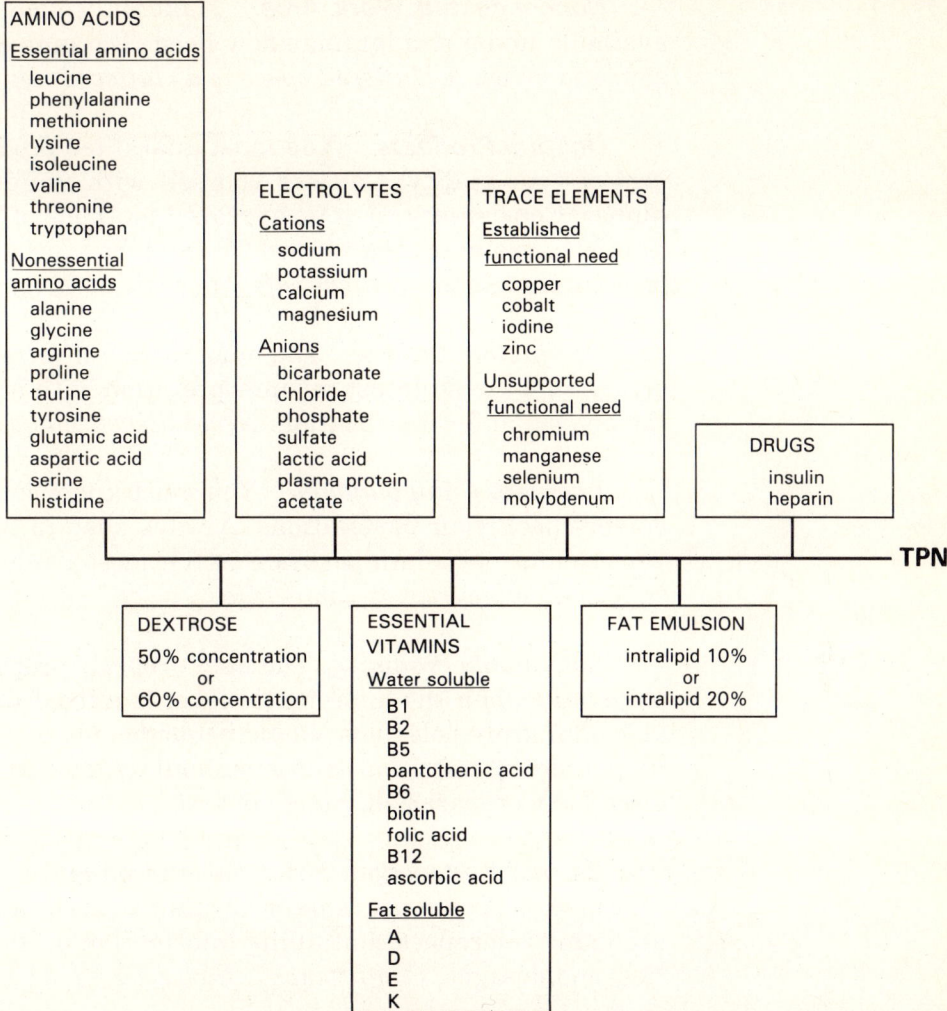

Figure 8-6 Elements of total parenteral nutrition.

you learn, and familiarity with the products you use will develop from experience. Regardless of the changes and advancements you encounter, some rules never change.

Rules for Proper Mixing

Aseptic Technique. Always follow the rules of aseptic technique. Use alcohol to cleanse and sterilize diaphragm tops of vials, laminar flow hood work spaces, and so on. Take every precaution to assure purity, safety, and sterility by preventing contamination. Intravenous solutions should always be prepared under a clean laminar flow hood. *Nothing can be substituted for cleanliness, care, and caution.*

Proper Mechanics. There is only a right way to prepare intravenous solutions and mixtures. Never substitute convenience and shortcuts for good judgment and accepted admixture preparation techniques. *Haste makes waste.*

Noncongested Work Area. Make only your needed accessories available under the laminar flow hood. Too many items invite confusion and error. *A cluttered space is a cluttered mind.*

Uniform Products. You must guarantee product integrity to the best of your ability. Concern yourself with uniformity in your techniques. Consistency in your approved methods of admixture preparation is a sure approach toward freedom from pyrogens, microbes, and particulate matter. *Patient safety is basic to the practice of pharmacy.*

Interpretive Orders. You must interpret intravenous orders properly. Avoid the slightest misinterpretation with a call to the prescribing physician for clarification. *Never dispense guesswork.*

Accurate Compounding. You must know your mathematics and double-check your calculations. Always keep in mind that the intravenous route of administration is the most dangerous route. *Knowledge is the precursor to competence.*

Acceptable Product. The final properly prepared product is complete only when the appropriate label is affixed to the bottle. Acceptable admixture solutions should be made only at the time of need. Total parenteral nutrition solutions should be discarded forty-eight hours after their preparation. *Safety is first.*

Current Knowledge. You have an obligation to be current with information. You must remain constant with the state of the art. There are many references containing information on safety, incompatibilities, and dosages. *Competence is the precursor to confidence.*

Hospital Policy. You must always be aware of hospital policy and hospital intravenous protocols. Protocols are usually the result of intense research and investigation used by pharmacy therapeutics committees. *What is proven is true.*

Self-protection. You should take every precaution to protect yourself from highly toxic drugs (that is, chemotherapeutic agents). Wear surgical gloves, masks, and proper smocks. Carefully change surgical gloves within each half hour. Properly dispose of used supplies. *Caution is an IV technician's best friend.*

INTRAVENOUS CALCULATIONS

The mathematics for calculating the necessary ingredients of an intravenous solution is fundamental. Ratio, proportion, and percentages are the essential areas of mathematics for providing safe and effective admixtures to patients.

In addition to patient safety, correct calculations assure product economy by minimizing product waste. You should start early to train yourself to be accurate, and assure your accuracy by always rechecking your numbers, calculations, and mathematical processes. If necessary, consult with the pharmacist or ask another technician to review your calculations. Be sure a pharmacist checks your final calculations and product.

Review the sample TPN solution order shown in Figure 8-7. Cover the answer. Using the available information, calculate the necessary volumes of each electrolyte, insulin, and heparin to be used.

Hardware

Specific IV hardware is used to prepare large volume infusion solutions. Likewise, additives used in admixtures and the reconstitution of many drugs require IV hardware.

Needles. Vary in diameter size (gauge) and length. The larger the gauge, the smaller the diameter. An eighteen-gauge needle has a smaller diameter than a sixteen-gauge needle.

Syringes. Vary in size and calibrations. Some syringes are specific for drugs given in small amounts or requiring specific calibrations such as insulin ("insulin" syringe) and tuberculin ("tuberculin" syringe).

Catheters. Must be sterile for the preparation of intravenous products. They vary in length and style (straight or "Y"-shaped).

Filters. Are necessary to filter particulate matter and materials usually greater than 0.22 microns in size.

Containers. Vary widely in composition (glass or plastic), content (drug, solution, evacuated, partial fill, frozen), and purpose (receptacle for admixture preparation, "piggyback," small volume drugs such as antibiotics, ready-for-use solutions).

Pump Infusions. Deliver accurate quantities and volumes of drugs in a rapid fashion. They usually require a syringe into which a solution is drawn.

Transfer Spikes. Enable the transfer of drugs reconstituted in a small vial to be added to large volume solutions. They are double-ended piercing pins. Some spikes are specialized, such as the *chemo dispensing pin*, used for chemotherapeutic medications.

Connectors. Used to assure proper closure between a catheter end and a syringe, needle, or another catheter. The most commonly used lock is known as the Luer lock.

Administration Sets. Used to transfer the many components (drugs, fluids, etc.) which often make up a final product. Sets include general sets, piggyback sets, filter sets, extension sets, transfer sets, and more.

TIPS

- Solutions should be clear (including colored solutions).
- Always check expiration dates of products being used.

MEMORIAL HOSPITAL
BALTIMORE, MARYLAND
PHYSICIAN'S ORDER RECORD

BEAR DOWN ON HARD SURFACE WITH BALL POINT PEN

PATIENT: John Doe
AGE: 47
SEX: M
RACE: Cauc.
CHART NO. 009876D

GENERIC EQUIVALENT IS AUTHORIZED UNLESS CHECKED IN THIS COLUMN

ALLERGY OR SENSITIVITY TO: NKDA
NONE KNOWN ☐ SIGNED: _____
DIAGNOSIS: S/P TUR

| DATE | TIME | ORDERS | PHYSICIAN'S SIG. |

TOTAL PARENTERAL NUTRITION (TPN) SOLUTION ORDERS—CENTRAL

AMINOSYN 10%   500 ml   Final Concentration 5%
DEXTROSE 50% WATER 500 ml   Final Concentration 25%
Rate **100** ml/hour

Bottle # **9**
POTASSIUM PHOSPHATE   10 mEq   OTHER _____
SODIUM CHLORIDE   **40** mEq   OTHER _____
SODIUM ACETATE   **20** mEq   HEPARIN   1000 UNITS
POTASSIUM CHLORIDE   **40** mEq   TRACE ELEMENTS *see below
REGULAR HUMULIN   **10** units VITAMINS   *see below

AMINOSYN 10%   500 ml   Final Concentration 5%
DEXTROSE 50%   500 ml   Final Concentration 25%
Rate **100** ml/hour

Bottle # **10** MULTI-ELECTROLYTE CONCENTRATE CONSISTING OF:
        SODIUM   25 mEq   CALCIUM   5 mEq   CHLORIDE 30 mEq
        POTASSIUM 20 mEq   MAGNESIUM   5 mEq   ACETATE   25 mEq
HEPARIN   1000 units
REGULAR HUMULIN   **8** units
OTHER APPROVED ADDITIVE _____

20% FAT EMULSION IS TO RUN CONTINUOUSLY THROUGH THE PROXIMAL MEDICINAL ENTRY AT 20 ml/hour (PHARMACY WILL SEQUENTIALLY LETTER BEGINNING WITH A)

NOTE: VITAMINS AND TRACE ELEMENTS WILL BE ADDED AS DESCRIBED IN PROTOCOL
Hang all bottles in consecutive order. RECORD the <u>EXACT TIME</u> hung as well as the bottle number and total volume. Maintain a constant rate. <u>DO NOT</u> catch up or slow down the infusion. Orders must be rewritten DAILY. THE TPN LINE SHOULD NOT BE USED FOR ANY OTHER PURPOSE.
PATIENTS ON TPN ARE TO RECEIVE:

1. CBC, BUN, LYTES, CREATININE, GLUCOSE every day for five days then MONDAYS and THURSDAYS.
2. SGOT, Ca, ALK PHOS, Mg, SGPT, BILIRUBIN, ALBUMIN, GLOBULIN, PO_4, PROTHROMBIN TIME, PARTIAL THROMBOPLASTIN TIME Monday, Thursday for the first week, then weekly.
3. Urine Acetone and Glucose and Specific Gravity every four hours for the first week then four times a day.
4. Weigh daily.
5. Serum transferrin level once per week.
6. In depleted patients and patients on prolonged hyperalimentation trace element levels should be requested.
7. Weekly twenty-four hour urine with an ALIQUOT for CREATININE and UREA NITROGEN.
8. DIETARY CONSULT.

PHARMACY COPY

Figure 8-7 Sample TPN order and calculations.

Intravenous Calculations

SUPPLIES:

Electrolyte/Drug	Abbreviation	How Supplied
potassium phosphate	KPO_4	10 ml. vial containing 4.4 mEq./ml.
sodium chloride	NaCl	30 ml. vial containing 4 mEq./ml.
sodium acetate	Na Acet.	20 ml. vial containing 40 mEq.
potassium chloride	KCl	10 ml. vial containing 20 mEq.
insulin		10 ml. vial containing 100 u/ml.
heparin		4 ml. vial containing 10,000 u/ml.

CALCULATIONS FOR BOTTLE #9:

Ingredient	Required Amount
KPO_4	10 mEq.

Solution: Each ml. of KPO_4 contains 4.4 mEq. Therefore, use 10 mEq./4.4 mEq. = 2.27 ml. 2.27 ml. provides 10 mEq.

Ingredient	Required Amount
NaCl	40 mEq.

Solution: Each ml. of NaCl contains 4 mEq. Therefore, use 40 mEq./4 mEq. = 10 ml. 10 ml. provides 40 mEq.

Ingredient	Required Amount
Na Acet.	20 mEq.

Solution: Each vial of Na Acet. contains 40 mEq. Therefore, use 20 mEq./40 mEq. = $\frac{1}{2}$ vial. $\frac{1}{2}$ of the 20 ml. vial is 10 ml. 10 ml. will contain 20 mEq. required.

Ingredient	Required Amount
KCl	40 mEq.

Solution: Each vial contains 20 mEq. Therefore, use 40 mEq./20 mEq. = 2 vials. Two vials will provide 40 mEq. of KCl required.

Ingredient	Required Amount
insulin	10 units

Solution: Each vial contains 100 u per milliliter. Therefore, use 10 u/100 u = 0.1 ml. 0.1 ml. provides 10 units of insulin.

Ingredient	Required Amount
heparin	1000 units

Solution: Each vial contains 10,000 u/ml. Therefore, use 1000 u/10,000 u = 0.1 ml. 0.1 ml. provides 1000 units of heparin.

Figure 8-7 (*Continued*)

- Follow intravenous protocols explicitly.
- Dextrose supplies 3.4 calories per gram.
- Fat supplies 9 calories per gram.
- Protein supplies 4 calories per gram.
- The formula for *osmolarity* is:

$$\text{mOsm/L} = 100(\text{AA\%}) + 50(\text{dextrose \%}) + \text{mEq./L.}$$

- Complete a preparation before leaving the workstation.
- Work well inside the laminar flow hood.
- Run the laminar flow hood for at least thirty minutes before preparing IV products.
- Rotate supplies to assure orderly flow of expiration dates.
- Have supplies readily available.
- Label, date, and properly store partially used vials.
- Know key abbreviations used in IV admixture programs and add to this list when necessary. See Table 8-3.

TABLE 8-3

Important Abbreviations Used in Intravenous Admixture Programs

Abbreviation	Meaning
AA	amino acids
IV or I.V.	intravenous
mEq.	milliequivalent
IVPB	intravenous piggyback
NS	normal saline
R	Ringer's solution
LR	Lactated Ringer's solution
Na Bicarb	sodium bicarbonate
Na lact	sodium lactate

IV pharmacy is perhaps the most challenging, demanding, and critical area of pharmacy. If you adhere to the proper principles associated with preparing IV products, you will easily meet the challenge and demand, thereby assuring your ultimate goal—safety to the patient and effectiveness of the therapy.

CALCULATIONS PRACTICE

Practice TPN Orders

Review the following practice TPN orders (Figures 8-8 to 8-11). Complete the calculations for each practice problem using the same format as in the sample order in Figure 8-7. Solutions may be found at the end of this chapter.

Calculations Practice

PATIENT: Jane Doe
AGE: 38
SEX: F
RACE: N
CHART NO. 002346J

MEMORIAL HOSPITAL
BALTIMORE, MARYLAND
PHYSICIAN'S ORDER RECORD

BEAR DOWN ON HARD SURFACE WITH BALL POINT PEN

GENERIC EQUIVALENT IS AUTHORIZED UNLESS CHECKED IN THIS COLUMN

ALLERGY OR SENSITIVITY TO: ASA
NONE KNOWN □ SIGNED: _(signature)_
DIAGNOSIS: S/P remove mass (R) lung

DATE	TIME	ORDERS	PHYSICIAN'S SIG.
	••		••

TOTAL PARENTERAL NUTRITION (TPN) SOLUTION ORDERS—CENTRAL

AMINOSYN 10%   500 ml   Final Concentration 5%
DEXTROSE 50% WATER 500 ml   Final Concentration 25%
Rate **100** ml/hour
Bottle # **12**
- POTASSIUM PHOSPHATE   10 mEq   OTHER _____
- SODIUM CHLORIDE   **40** mEq   OTHER _____
- SODIUM ACETATE   ___ mEq   HEPARIN   1000 UNITS
- POTASSIUM CHLORIDE   **50** mEq   TRACE ELEMENTS *see below
- REGULAR HUMULIN   ___ units   VITAMINS   *see below

AMINOSYN 10%   500 ml   Final Concentration 5%
DEXTROSE 50%   500 ml   Final Concentration 25%
Rate **100** ml/hour
Bottle # **13** MULTI-ELECTROLYTE CONCENTRATE CONSISTING OF:
- SODIUM 25 mEq   CALCIUM 5 mEq   CHLORIDE 30 mEq
- POTASSIUM 20 mEq   MAGNESIUM 5 mEq   ACETATE 25 mEq
- HEPARIN   1000 units
- REGULAR HUMULIN   **10** units
- OTHER APPROVED ADDITIVE _____

20% FAT EMULSION IS TO RUN CONTINUOUSLY THROUGH THE PROXIMAL MEDICINAL ENTRY AT 20 ml/hour (PHARMACY WILL SEQUENTIALLY LETTER BEGINNING WITH A)

NOTE: VITAMINS AND TRACE ELEMENTS WILL BE ADDED AS DESCRIBED IN PROTOCOL
Hang all bottles in consecutive order. RECORD the EXACT TIME hung as well as the bottle number and total volume. Maintain a constant rate. DO NOT catch up or slow down the infusion. Orders must be rewritten DAILY. THE TPN LINE SHOULD NOT BE USED FOR ANY OTHER PURPOSE.
PATIENTS ON TPN ARE TO RECEIVE:

1. CBC, BUN, LYTES, CREATININE, GLUCOSE every day for five days then MONDAYS and THURSDAYS.
2. SGOT, Ca, ALK PHOS, Mg, SGPT, BILIRUBIN, ALBUMIN, GLOBULIN, PO_4, PROTHROMBIN TIME, PARTIAL THROMBOPLASTIN TIME Monday, Thursday for the first week, then weekly.
3. Urine Acetone and Glucose and Specific Gravity every four hours for the first week then four times a day.
4. Weigh daily.
5. Serum transferrin level once per week.
6. In depleted patients and patients on prolonged hyperalimentation trace element levels should be requested.
7. Weekly twenty-four hour urine with an ALIQUOT for CREATININE and UREA NITROGEN.
8. DIETARY CONSULT.

PHARMACY COPY

Figure 8-8

MEMORIAL HOSPITAL
BALTIMORE, MARYLAND
PHYSICIAN'S ORDER RECORD

BEAR DOWN ON HARD SURFACE WITH BALL POINT PEN

PATIENT: Jim Doe
AGE: 53
SEX: M
RACE: Cauc.
CHART NO. 001357JD

GENERIC EQUIVALENT IS AUTHORIZED UNLESS CHECKED IN THIS COLUMN

ALLERGY OR SENSITIVITY TO: ∅
NONE KNOWN ☐ SIGNED: _(signature)_

DIAGNOSIS: Intestinal Obstruction

DATE	TIME	ORDERS	PHYSICIAN'S SIG.

TOTAL PARENTERAL NUTRITION (TPN) SOLUTION ORDERS—CENTRAL

AMINOSYN 10%   500 ml   Final Concentration 5%
DEXTROSE 50% WATER   500 ml   Final Concentration 25%
Rate **100** ml/hour

Bottle # **4**
- POTASSIUM PHOSPHATE   10 mEq   OTHER _____
- SODIUM CHLORIDE   **40** mEq OTHER _____
- SODIUM ACETATE   **40** mEq HEPARIN 1000 UNITS
- POTASSIUM CHLORIDE   ___ mEq   TRACE ELEMENTS *see below
- REGULAR HUMULIN   ___ units   VITAMINS *see below

AMINOSYN 10%   500 ml   Final Concentration 5%
DEXTROSE 50%   500 ml   Final Concentration 25%
Rate **100** ml/hour

Bottle # **5**   MULTI-ELECTROLYTE CONCENTRATE CONSISTING OF:
- SODIUM 25 mEq   CALCIUM 5 mEq   CHLORIDE 30 mEq
- POTASSIUM 20 mEq MAGNESIUM 5 mEq ACETATE 25 mEq
- HEPARIN   1000 units
- REGULAR HUMULIN   **8** units
- OTHER APPROVED ADDITIVE _____

20% FAT EMULSION IS TO RUN CONTINUOUSLY THROUGH THE PROXIMAL MEDICINAL ENTRY AT 20 ml/hour (PHARMACY WILL SEQUENTIALLY LETTER BEGINNING WITH A)

NOTE: VITAMINS AND TRACE ELEMENTS WILL BE ADDED AS DESCRIBED IN PROTOCOL
Hang all bottles in consecutive order. RECORD the <u>EXACT TIME</u> hung as well as the bottle number and total volume. Maintain a constant rate. <u>DO NOT</u> catch up or slow down the infusion. Orders must be rewritten <u>DAILY. THE TPN LINE SHOULD NOT BE USED FOR ANY OTHER PURPOSE.</u>
<u>PATIENTS ON TPN ARE TO RECEIVE:</u>

1. CBC, BUN, LYTES, CREATININE, GLUCOSE every day for five days then MONDAYS and THURSDAYS.
2. SGOT, Ca, ALK PHOS, Mg, SGPT, BILIRUBIN, ALBUMIN, GLOBULIN, PO$_4$, PROTHROMBIN TIME, PARTIAL THROMBOPLASTIN TIME Monday, Thursday for the first week, then weekly.
3. Urine Acetone and Glucose and Specific Gravity every four hours for the first week then four times a day.
4. Weigh daily.
5. Serum transferrin level once per week.
6. In depleted patients and patients on prolonged hyperalimentation trace element levels should be requested.
7. Weekly twenty-four hour urine with an ALIQUOT for CREATININE and UREA NITROGEN.
8. DIETARY CONSULT.

PHARMACY COPY

Figure 8-9

Calculations Practice 143

PATIENT: Liu Doe	MEMORIAL HOSPITAL
AGE: 60	BALTIMORE, MARYLAND
SEX: M	PHYSICIAN'S ORDER RECORD
RACE: Oriental	
CHART NO. 002468DL	BEAR DOWN ON HARD SURFACE WITH BALL POINT PEN

GENERIC EQUIVALENT IS AUTHORIZED UNLESS CHECKED IN THIS COLUMN

ALLERGY OR SENSITIVITY TO: Ragweed, fish
NONE KNOWN ☐ SIGNED: [signature]
DIAGNOSIS: ABD. CA.

DATE	TIME	ORDERS	PHYSICIAN'S SIG.
		••	••

TOTAL PARENTERAL NUTRITION (TPN) SOLUTION ORDERS—CENTRAL

AMINOSYN 10%   500 ml   Final Concentration 5%
DEXTROSE 50% WATER 500 ml   Final Concentration 25%
Rate **100** ml/hour
Bottle # **11**   POTASSIUM PHOSPHATE 10 mEq   OTHER _____
                  SODIUM CHLORIDE   **80** mEq   OTHER _____
                  SODIUM ACETATE   ____ mEq   HEPARIN 1000 UNITS
                  POTASSIUM CHLORIDE ____ mEq   TRACE ELEMENTS *see below
                  REGULAR HUMULIN   ____ units VITAMINS   *see below

AMINOSYN 10%   500 ml   Final Concentration 5%
DEXTROSE 50%   500 ml   Final Concentration 25%
Rate **100** ml/hour
Bottle # **12**   MULTI-ELECTROLYTE CONCENTRATE CONSISTING OF:
                  SODIUM   25 mEq   CALCIUM   5 mEq   CHLORIDE 30 mEq
                  POTASSIUM   20 mEq   MAGNESIUM 5 mEq   ACETATE 25 mEq
                  HEPARIN   1000 units
                  REGULAR HUMULIN   ____ units
                  OTHER APPROVED ADDITIVE _____

20% FAT EMULSION IS TO RUN CONTINUOUSLY THROUGH THE PROXIMAL MEDICINAL ENTRY AT 20 ml/hour (PHARMACY WILL SEQUENTIALLY LETTER BEGINNING WITH A)

NOTE: VITAMINS AND TRACE ELEMENTS WILL BE ADDED AS DESCRIBED IN PROTOCOL
Hang all bottles in consecutive order. RECORD the EXACT TIME hung as well as the bottle number and total volume. Maintain a constant rate. DO NOT catch up or slow down the infusion. Orders must be rewritten DAILY. THE TPN LINE SHOULD NOT BE USED FOR ANY OTHER PURPOSE.
PATIENTS ON TPN ARE TO RECEIVE:

1. CBC, BUN, LYTES, CREATININE, GLUCOSE every day for five days then MONDAYS and THURSDAYS.
2. SGOT, Ca, ALK PHOS, Mg, SGPT, BILIRUBIN, ALBUMIN, GLOBULIN, PO_4, PROTHROMBIN TIME, PARTIAL THROMBOPLASTIN TIME Monday, Thursday for the first week, then weekly.
3. Urine Acetone and Glucose and Specific Gravity every four hours for the first week then four times a day.
4. Weigh daily.
5. Serum transferrin level once per week.
6. In depleted patients and patients on prolonged hyperalimentation trace element levels should be requested.
7. Weekly twenty-four hour urine with an ALIQUOT for CREATININE and UREA NITROGEN.
8. DIETARY CONSULT.

PHARMACY COPY

Figure 8-10

Chap. 8 / Intravenous Pharmacy

MEMORIAL HOSPITAL
BALTIMORE, MARYLAND
PHYSICIAN'S ORDER RECORD

BEAR DOWN ON HARD SURFACE WITH BALL POINT PEN

PATIENT: Jennifer Doe
AGE: 33
SEX: F
RACE: Cauc.
CHART NO. 009753DJ

GENERIC EQUIVALENT IS AUTHORIZED UNLESS CHECKED IN THIS COLUMN

ALLERGY OR SENSITIVITY
TO _____
NONE KNOWN [X]   SIGNED: _____

DIAGNOSIS: Toxic Colitis / SP colectomy

DATE	TIME	ORDERS	PHYSICIAN'S SIG.

TOTAL PARENTERAL NUTRITION (TPN) SOLUTION ORDERS—CENTRAL

AMINOSYN 10%   500 ml   Final Concentration 5%
DEXTROSE 50% WATER 500 ml   Final Concentration 25%
Rate **100** ml/hour
Bottle # **14**
  POTASSIUM PHOSPHATE   10 mEq   OTHER _____
  SODIUM CHLORIDE   **40** mEq OTHER _____
  SODIUM ACETATE   **20** mEq HEPARIN   1000 UNITS
  POTASSIUM CHLORIDE   **20** mEq TRACE ELEMENTS *see below
  REGULAR HUMULIN   ___ units   VITAMINS   *see below

AMINOSYN 10%   500 ml   Final Concentration 5%
DEXTROSE 50%   500 ml   Final Concentration 25%
Rate **100** ml/hour
Bottle # **15** MULTI-ELECTROLYTE CONCENTRATE CONSISTING OF:
            SODIUM   25 mEq   CALCIUM   5 mEq   CHLORIDE 30 mEq
            POTASSIUM 20 mEq   MAGNESIUM 5 mEq   ACETATE 25 mEq
  HEPARIN   1000 units
  REGULAR HUMULIN ___ units
  OTHER APPROVED ADDITIVE _____

20% FAT EMULSION IS TO RUN CONTINUOUSLY THROUGH THE PROXIMAL MEDICINAL ENTRY AT 20 ml/hour (PHARMACY WILL SEQUENTIALLY LETTER BEGINNING WITH A)

NOTE: VITAMINS AND TRACE ELEMENTS WILL BE ADDED AS DESCRIBED IN PROTOCOL
Hang all bottles in consecutive order. RECORD the EXACT TIME hung as well as the bottle number and total volume. Maintain a constant rate. DO NOT catch up or slow down the infusion. Orders must be rewritten DAILY. THE TPN LINE SHOULD NOT BE USED FOR ANY OTHER PURPOSE.
PATIENTS ON TPN ARE TO RECEIVE:

1. CBC, BUN, LYTES, CREATININE, GLUCOSE every day for five days then MONDAYS and THURSDAYS.
2. SGOT, Ca, ALK PHOS, Mg, SGPT, BILIRUBIN, ALBUMIN, GLOBULIN, PO4, PROTHROMBIN TIME, PARTIAL THROMBOPLASTIN TIME Monday, Thursday for the first week, then weekly.
3. Urine Acetone and Glucose and Specific Gravity every four hours for the first week then four times a day.
4. Weigh daily.
5. Serum transferrin level once per week.
6. In depleted patients and patients on prolonged hyperalimentation trace element levels should be requested.
7. Weekly twenty-four hour urine with an ALIQUOT for CREATININE and UREA NITROGEN.
8. DIETARY CONSULT.

PHARMACY COPY

Figure 8-11

Calculations Practice

Solutions

The SUPPLIES are the same for all the practice TPN orders:

Electrolyte/Drug	Abbreviation	How Supplied
potassium phosphate	KPO_4	10 ml. vial containing 4.4 mEq./ml.
sodium chloride	NaCl	30 ml. vial containing 4 mEq./ml.
sodium acetate	Na Acet.	20 ml. vial containing 40 mEq.
potassium chloride	KCl	10 ml. vial containing 20 mEq.
insulin		10 ml. vial containing 100 u/ml.
heparin		4 ml. vial containing 10,000 u/ml.

Figure 8-8

CALCULATIONS FOR BOTTLE #12:

Ingredient	Required Amount	Solution
KPO_4	10 mEq.	10 mEq./4.4 mEq. = x ml./1 ml. x = 2.27 ml.
NaCl	40 mEq.	40 mEq./4 mEq. = x ml./1 ml. x = 10.0 ml. ($\frac{1}{3}$ of the vial)
KCl	50 mEq.	50 mEq./20 mEq. = x ml./10 ml. x = 25.0 ml. ($2\frac{1}{2}$ vials)

CALCULATIONS FOR BOTTLE #13:

Ingredient	Required Amount	Solution
insulin	10 u	10 u/100 u = x ml./1 ml. x = 0.1 ml.

Figure 8-9

CALCULATIONS FOR BOTTLE #4:

Ingredient	Required Amount	Solution
KPO_4	10 mEq.	10 mEq./4.4 mEq. = x ml./1 ml. x = 2.27 ml.
NaCl	40 mEq.	40 mEq./4 mEq. = x ml./1 ml. x = 10 ml. ($\frac{1}{3}$ of the vial)
Na Acet.	40 mEq.	40 mEq./40 mEq. = x ml./20 ml. x = 20 ml. (1 vial)

CALCULATIONS FOR BOTTLE #5:

Ingredient	Required Amount	Solution
insulin	8 u	8 u/100 u = x ml./1 ml. x = 0.08 ml.

Figure 8-10

CALCULATIONS FOR BOTTLE #11:

Ingredient	Required Amount	Solution
KPO_4	10 mEq.	10 mEq./4.4 mEq. = x ml./1 ml. x = 2.27 ml.
NaCl	80 mEq.	80 mEq./4 mEq. = x ml./1 ml. x = 20 ml. ($\frac{2}{3}$ of the vial)

CALCULATIONS FOR BOTTLE #12:
No calculations are required

Figure 8-11

CALCULATIONS FOR BOTTLE #14:

Ingredient	Required Amount	Solution
KPO_4	10 mEq.	10 mEq./4.4 mEq. = x ml./1 ml. x = 2.27 ml.
NaCl	40 mEq.	40 mEq./4 mEq. = x ml./1 ml. x = 10 ml. ($\frac{1}{3}$ of the vial)
Na Acet.	20 mEq.	20 mEq./40 mEq. = x ml./20 ml. x = 10 ml. ($\frac{1}{2}$ of the vial)
KCl	20 mEq.	20 mEq./20 mEq. = x ml./10 ml. x = 10 ml. (1 vial)

CALCULATIONS FOR BOTTLE #15:
No calculations are required

APPENDIX A

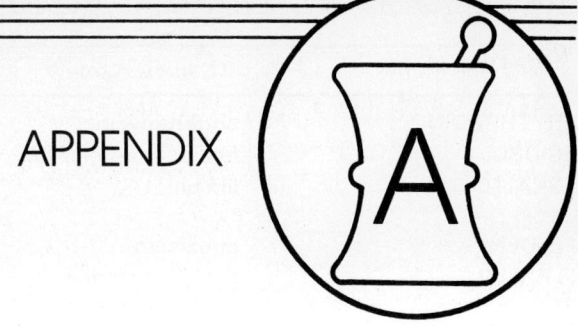

Trade and Generic Names of Common Drugs

Trade Name	Generic Name
ACHROMYCIN V	tetracycline
ADAPIN	doxepin
ALDACTONE	spironolactone
ALDOMET	methyldopa
ALUPENT	metaproterenol
AMCILL	ampicillin
AMOXIL	amoxicillin
ANAPROX	naproxen
APRESOLINE	hydralazine
ATARAX	hydroxyzine
ATIVAN	lorazepam
BACTRIM	co-trimoxazole
BEEPEN VK	penicillin VK
BENADRYL	diphenhydramine
BENEMID	probenecid
BENTYL	dicyclomine
BLOCADREN	timolol
BRETHINE	terbutaline
BUMEX	bumetanide
CALAN	verapamil
CAPOTEN	captopril
CARAFATE	sucralfate
CARDIZEM	diltiazem
CATAPRES	clonidine

Trade Name	Generic Name
CECLOR	cefaclor
CENTRAX	prazepam
CLEOCIN	clindamycin
CLINORIL	sulindac
COGENTIN	benztropine
CORGARD	nadolol
COUMADIN	warfarin
DALMANE	flurazepam
DELTASONE	prednisone
DESYREL	trazodone
DIABETA	glyburide
DIABINESE	chlorpropamide
DILANTIN	phenytoin
DITROPAN	oxybutynin
DIURIL	chlorothiazide
DOLOBID	diflunisal
DURICEF	cefadroxil
DYMELOR	acetohexamide
DYRENIUM	triamterene
E.E.S.	erythromycin
E-MYCIN	erythromycin
ELAVIL	amitriptyline
ENDURON	methyclothiazide
ERYC	erythromycin

Trade Name	Generic Name	Trade Name	Generic Name
ERYTHROCIN	erythromycin	MICRONASE	glyburide
ESIDRIX	hydrochlorothiazide	MIDAMOR	amiloride
ESKALITH	lithium	MINIPRESS	prazosin
		MINOCIN	minocycline
FELDENE	piroxicam	MONISTAT	miconazole
FLEXERIL	cyclobenzaprine	MOTRIN	ibuprofen
		MYSOLINE	primidone
GARAMYCIN	gentamicin		
GLUCOTROL	glypizide	NALFON	fenoprofen
		NAPROSYN	naproxen
HALCION	triazolam	NASALIDE	flunisolide
HALDOL	haloperidol	NATURETIN	bendroflumethiazide
HYDERGINE	ergoloids	NAVANE	thiothixene
HYDRODIURIL	hydrochlorothiazide	NEPTAZANE	methazolamide
HYGROTON	chlorthalidone	NICORETTE	nicotine
HYTONE	hydrocortisone	NITRO-BID	nitroglycerine
		NITRO-DUR	nitroglycerine
ILOSONE	erythromycin	NITROSTAT	nitroglycerine
IMODIUM	loperamide	NOLVADEX	tamoxifen
INH	isoniazid	NORMODYNE	labetalol
INDERAL	propranolol	NORPACE	disopyramide
INDOCIN	indomethacin	NORPRAMIN	desipramine
INTAL	cromolyn		
ISOPTIN	verapamil	OGEN	estrone
ISORDIL	isosorbide	OMNIPEN	ampicillin
		ORINASE	tolbutamide
K-LYTE	potassium		
K-TAB	potassium	PEN VEE K	penicillin VK
KAON	potassium	PERSANTINE	dipyridamole
KEFLEX	cephalexin	PHENERGAN	promethazine
KLOTRIX	potassium	POLYCILLIN	ampicillin
		POLYMOX	amoxicillin
LANOXIN	digoxin	PREMARIN	conjugated estrogens
LAROTID	amoxicillin	PRINCIPEN	ampicillin
LASIX	furosemide	PROCAN	procainamide
LEDERCILLIN VK	penicillin VK	PROCARDIA	nifedipine
LEVOTHROID	levothyroxine	PROVENTIL	albuterol
LIBRIUM	chlordiazepoxide	PROVERA	medroxyprogesterone
LIDEX	flucinolone		
LOPID	gemfibrozil	QUINAGLUTE DURA-TABS	quinidine
LOPRESSOR	metoprolol	QUINAMM	quinine
LOPURIN	allopurinol	QUINIDEX	quinidine
LOTRIMIN	clotrimazole		
LOZOL	indapamide	REGLAN	metoclopramide
LUDIOMIL	maprotiline	RENESE	polythiazide
LUMINAL	phenobarbital	RESTORIL	temazepam
		RETIN-A	tretinoin
MACRODANTIN	nitrofurantoin	RITALIN	methylphenidate
MECLOMEN	meclofenamate	RUFEN	ibuprofen
MEDROL	methylprednisone		
MELLARIL	thioridazine	SELDANE	terfenadine
METAHYDRIN	trichlormethiazide	SEPTRA	co-trimoxazole
MICRO-K	potassium	SERAX	oxazepam

App. A / Trade and Generic Names of Common Drugs

Trade Name	Generic Name
SERPASIL	reserpine
SINEQUAN	doxepin
SLO-BID	theophylline
SLOW-K	potassium
SLO-PHYLLIN	theophylline
SORBITRATE	isosorbide
SUMYCIN	tetracycline
SYNTHROID	levothyroxine
TAGAMET	cimetidine
TALWIN NX	pentazocine
TAVIST	clemastine
TEGRETOL	carbamazepine
TENORMIN	atenolol
THEO-DUR	theophylline
THYRAR	thyroid
TIMOPTIC	timolol
TOLECTIN	tolmetin
TOLINASE	tolazamide
TOPICORT	desoximetasone
TRANSDERM-NITRO	nitroglycerine
TRANXENE	clorazepate
TRENTAL	pentoxifylline
TRINALIN	azatadine

Trade Name	Generic Name
V-CILLIN K	penicillin VK
VALISONE	betamethasone
VALIUM	diazepam
VANCERIL	beclomethasone
VASOTEC	enalapril
VEETIDS	penicillin V
VENTOLIN	albuterol
VIBRAMYCIN	doxycycline
VIBRA-TABS	doxycycline
VISKEN	pindolol
VISTARIL	hydroxyzine
WYMOX	amoxicillin
WYTENSIN	guanabenz
XANAX	alprazolam
ZANTAC	ranitidine
ZAROXOLYN	metolazone
ZOVIRAX	acyclovir
ZYLOPRIM	allopurinol

Generic Name	Trade Name
acetaminophen	TYLENOL
acetohexamide	DYMELOR
acyclovir	ZOVIRAX
albuterol	PROVENTIL, VENTOLIN
allopurinol	ZYLOPRIM, LOPURIN
alprazolam	XANAX
amiloride	MIDAMOR
amitriptyline	ELAVIL
amoxicillin	AMOXIL, POLYMOX, WYMOX, LAROTID
ampicillin	POLYCILLIN, OMNIPEN, AMCILL, PRINCIPEN
atenolol	TENORMIN
azatadine	TRINALIN
beclomethasone	VANCERIL
bendroflumethiazide	NATURETIN
benztropine	COGENTIN
betamethasone	VALISONE
bumetanide	BUMEX
captopril	CAPOTEN
carbamazepine	TEGRETOL
cefaclor	CECLOR
cefadroxil	DURICEF

Generic Name	Trade Name
cephalexin	KEFLEX
chlordiazepoxide	LIBRIUM
chlorothiazide	DIURIL
chlorpropamide	DIABENESE
chlorthalidone	HYGROTON
cimetidine	TAGAMET
clemastine	TAVIST
clindamycin	CLEOCIN
clonidine	CATAPRES
clorazepate	TRANXENE
clotrimazole	LOTRIMIN
conjugated estrogens	PREMARIN
co-trimoxazole	BACTRIM, SEPTRA
cromolyn	INTAL
cyclobenzaprine	FLEXERIL
desipramine	NORPRAMIN
desoximetasone	TOPICORT
diazepam	VALIUM
dicyclomine	BENTYL
diflunisal	DOLOBID
digoxin	LANOXIN
diltiazem	CARDIZEM
diphenhydramine	BENADRYL

Generic Name	Trade Name
dipyridamole	PERSANTINE
disopyramide	NORPACE
doxepin	SINEQUAN, ADAPIN
doxycycline	VIBRA-TABS, VIRBRAMYCIN
enalapril	VASOTEC
ergoloids	HYDERGINE
erythromycin	E.E.S., E-MYCIN, ERYC, ERYTHROCIN, ILOSONE
estrone	OGEN
fenoprofen	NALFON
flucinolone	LIDEX
flunisolide	NASALIDE
flurazepam	DALMANE
furosemide	LASIX
gemfibrozil	LOPID
gentamicin	GARAMYCIN
glyburide	MICRONASE, DIABETA
glypizide	GLUCOTROL
guanabenz	WYTENSIN
haloperidol	HALDOL
hydralazine	APRESOLINE
hydrochlorothiazide	HYDRODIURIL, ESIDRIX
hydrocortisone	HYTONE
hydroxyzine	ATARAX, VISTARIL
ibuprofen	MOTRIN, RUFEN
indapamide	LOZOL
indomethacin	INDOCIN
isoniazid	INH
isosorbide	ISORDIL, SORBITRATE
labetalol	NORMODYNE
levothyroxine	SYNTHROID, LEVOTHROID
lithium	ESKALITH
loperamide	IMODIUM
lorazepam	ATIVAN
maprotiline	LUDIOMIL
meclofenamate	MECLOMEN
medroxyprogesterone	PROVERA
metaproterenol	ALUPENT
methazolamide	NEPTAZANE
methyclothiazide	ENDURON
methyldopa	ALDOMET
methylphenidate	RITALIN
methylprednisolone	MEDROL
metoclopramide	REGLAN
metolazone	ZAROXOLYN
metoprolol	LOPRESSOR
miconazole	MONISTAT
minocycline	MINOCIN
nadolol	CORGARD
naproxen	NAPROSYN, ANAPROX
nicotine	NICORETTE
nifedipine	PROCARDIA
nitrofurantoin	MACRODANTIN
nitroglycerine	NITROSTAT, TRANSDERM-NITRO, NITRO-BID, NITRO-DUR
oxazepam	SERAX
oxybutynin	DITROPAN
penicillin V	VEETIDS
penicillin VK	LEDERCILLIN VK, PEN VEE K, BEEPEN VK, V-CILLIN K
pentazocine	TALWIN NX
pentoxifylline	TRENTAL
phenobarbital	LUMINAL
phenytoin	DILANTIN
pindolol	VISKEN
piroxicam	FELDENE
polythiazide	RENESE
potassium	SLOW-K, MICRO-K, K-TAB, KLOTRIX, K-LYTE, KAON
prazepam	CENTRAX
prazosin	MINIPRESS
prednisone	DELTASONE
primidone	MYSOLINE
probenecid	BENEMID
procainamide	PROCAN
prochlorperazine	COMPAZINE
promethazine	PHENERGAN
propranolol	INDERAL
quinidine	QUINAGLUTE, DURA-TABS, QUINIDEX
quinine	QUINAMM
ranitidine	ZANTAC
reserpine	SERPASIL
spironolactone	ALDACTONE
sucralfate	CARAFATE
sulindac	CLINORIL
tamoxifen	NOLVADEX
temazepam	RESTORIL
terbutaline	BRETHINE

Generic Name	Trade Name	Generic Name	Trade Name
terfenadine	SELDANE	tolmetin	TOLECTIN
tetracycline	ACHROMYCIN V, SUMYCIN	trazodone	DESYREL
		tretinoin	RETIN-A
theophylline	THEO-DUR, SLO-BID, SLO-PHYLLIN	triamterene	DYRENIUM
		triazolam	HALCION
thioridazine	MELLARIL	trichlormethiazide	METAHYDRIN
thiothixene	NAVANE		
thyroid	THYRAR	verapamil	CALAN, ISOPTIN
timolol	TIMOPTIC, BLOCADREN		
tolazamide	TOLINASE		
tolbutamide	ORINASE	warfarin	COUMADIN

APPENDIX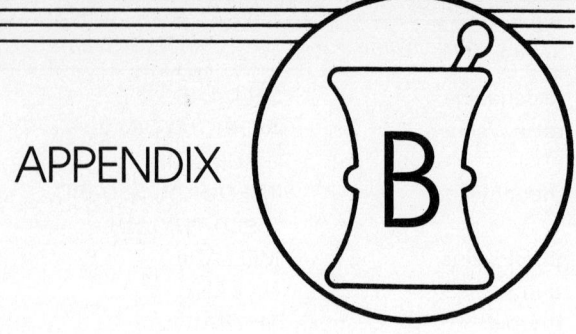

Common Drug Interactions

The drug interactions listed in this appendix were discovered, documented, and substantiated to be clinically significant.

Alcohol

produces an additive sedation with:

clonidine	anticonvulsants
methyldopa	antihistamines
reserpine	skeletal muscle relaxants
narcotic analgesics	sedative/hypnotics
psychotherapeutic agents	

produces additive gastric irritation with:

    salicylates

produces flushing, sweating, nausea and tachycardia with:

    chlorpropamide
    metronidazole
    cephalosporins

Anticoagulants, oral

have enhanced anticoagulant activity with:

amiodarone	phenylbutazone
aspirin	sulfinpyrazone
chloral hydrate	anabolic steroids
cimetidine	salicylates

clofibrate
metronidazole
sulfonamides
thyroid hormones

have reduced anticoagulant activity with:

carbamazepine
cholestyramine
glutethimide
griseofulvin
phytonadione
rifampin
barbiturates

Digitalis Glycosides (for example, digoxin)

have reduced bioavailability of drug with:

cholestyramine
colestipol
kaolin
neomycin
penicillamine
antacids

have enhanced cardiotoxic potential with:

amphotericin B
amiodarone
erythromycin base
quinidine
tetracycline
verapamil
corticosteroids
thiazide diuretics
loop diuretics

Doxycycline

has diminished effect with:

carbamazepine
phenobarbital
phenytoin

Guanethidine

has reduced antihypertensive effect with:

chlorpromazine
sympathomimetic amines
tricyclic antidepressants

Indomethacin

reduces the antihypertensive effects of:

captopril
beta blockers

Insulin

has enhanced hypoglycemic activity with:

propranolol
monoamine oxidase (MAO)
   inhibitors

Lidocaine

has enhanced potential for toxicity with:
- cimetidine
- propranolol

Lithium

has abnormal serum concentrations with:
- probenecid
- theophylline
- thiazide diuretics
- nonsteroidal anti-inflammatory agents (NSAIA)

Metoprolol or Propranolol

has enhanced activity with:
- chlorpromazine
- cimetidine
- oral contraceptives

has reduced activity with:
- rifamfin
- barbiturates

Oral Contraceptives

have reduced contraceptive activity with:
- phenytoin
- primidone
- ampicillin
- tetracycline
- barbiturates

Phenytoin

has increased serum concentration with:
- chloramphenicol
- cimetidine
- dicumarol
- isoniazid
- phenylbutazone
- trimethoprim
- sulfonamides

Quinidine

has enhanced activity with:
- amiodarone
- cimetidine

has reduced activity with:
- phenytoin
- rifampin
- barbiturates

Sulfonylureas

have enhanced hypoglycemic activity with:
- chloramphenicol
- dicumarol
- phenylbutazone
- clofibrate
- sulfonamides
- salicylates

Tetracyclines

have decreased bioavailability with:
- antacids
- calcium compounds
- iron compounds
- magnesium compounds

Theophylline

has enhanced activity with:
- cimetidine
- erythromycin

has reduced effect with:
- nadolol
- pindolol
- propranolol
- timolol
- phenytoin

Others

- Clonidine and propranolol can result in a rebound hypertension.
- Heparin and aspirin can result in enhanced anticoagulant activity.
- Meperidine and MAO inhibitors can result in enhanced central nervous system toxicity with symptoms such as excitation and convulsions.
- Methotrexate and salicylates or probenecid can result in an increased serum concentration of methotrexate.
- MAO inhibitors and ephedrine can result in hypertension.
- Phenobarbital and valproic acid can result in an increased serum concentration of phenobarbital.
- Primidone and phenytoin can result in increased primidone activity.
- Probenecid and salicylates can result in reduced antigout action of probenecid.
- Sulfinpyrazone and salicylates can result in reduced antigout activity of sulfinpyrazone.

APPENDIX

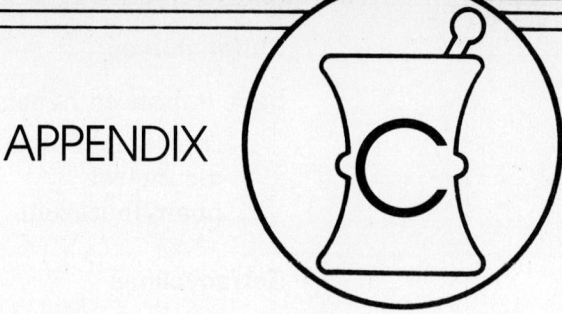

Practice Prescriptions

Review each of the following practice prescriptions (Figures C-1 to C-26). For each drug, give the *generic name*, the *trade name*, *strength*, *dosage form*, the *amount* to be *dispensed*, and the *directions to the patient*. Answers may be found following the prescriptions.

App. C / Practice Prescriptions 157

PAT SMITH, M.D.
27 Oak Leaf Lane
Baltimore, MD 12121
Phone: 322-7890

Name _____

Address _____

Age _____

℞ Lotrimin 1% Cream
15 Gm
Sig. apply to affected area BID
in AM & PM

[ ] Contents are labeled
unless checked

May be refilled 0 1 2 3 4

Signed _____ M.D.

Date _____ 19 ___ DEA No. _____

Figure C-1

PAT SMITH, M.D.
27 Oak Leaf Lane
Baltimore, MD 12121
Phone: 322-7890

Name _____

Address _____

Age _____

℞ Transderm-Nitro Patch
5 cm² (2.5 mg/24H)
#30
Sig. i q 24°

[ ] Contents are labeled
unless checked

May be refilled 0 1 2 3 4

Signed _____ M.D.

Date _____ 19 ___ DEA No. _____

Figure C-2

App. C / Practice Prescriptions

PAT SMITH, M.D.
27 Oak Leaf Lane
Baltimore, MD 12121
Phone: 322-7890

Name_____

Address_____

Age_____

℞ Timoptic 0.25%
  Ophthalmic drops
  #1
  S. gtts ī o.u. BID

[ ] Contents are labeled unless checked

May be refilled 0 1 2 3 4

Signed_____ M.D.

Date_____ 19___ DEA No._____

Figure C-3

PAT SMITH, M.D.
27 Oak Leaf Lane
Baltimore, MD 12121
Phone: 322-7890

Name_____

Address_____

Age_____

℞ Alupent Metered Dose (225mg)
  #1
  Inhale ii puffs q 3-4°
  No more than 12 per day

[ ] Contents are labeled unless checked

May be refilled 0 1 2 3 4

Signed_____ M.D.

Date_____ 19___ DEA No._____

Figure C-4

App. C / Practice Prescriptions 159

PAT SMITH, M.D.
27 Oak Leaf Lane
Baltimore, MD 12121
Phone: 322-7890

Name_____

Address_____

Age_____

℞ Caps Lopid 300 mg
#C
ii ½ h ā breakfast, ii ½ h ā dinner

[ ] Contents are labeled
unless checked

May be refilled 0 1 2 3 4

Signed_____ M.D.

Date_____ 19____ DEA No._____

Figure C-5

PAT SMITH, M.D.
27 Oak Leaf Lane
Baltimore, MD 12121
Phone: 322-7890

Name_____

Address_____

Age_____

℞ Premarin Tabs 1.25 mg
#40
i AM & PM for 20 d, rest 10 d,
resume schedule. Dispense
PPI

[ ] Contents are labeled
unless checked

May be refilled 0 1 2 3 4

Signed_____ M.D.

Date_____ 19____ DEA No._____

Figure C-6

App. C / Practice Prescriptions

PAT SMITH, M.D.
27 Oak Leaf Lane
Baltimore, MD 12121
Phone: 322-7890

Name _____
Address _____
Age _____

℞ Inderal 40mg
    #50
    S. 80mg daily (ī AM and ī PM)

[ ] Contents are labeled
    unless checked

May be refilled 0 1 2 3 4

Signed _____ M.D.
Date _____ 19___ DEA No. _____

Figure C-7

PAT SMITH, M.D.
27 Oak Leaf Lane
Baltimore, MD 12121
Phone: 322-7890

Name _____
Address _____
Age _____

℞ Synthroid 100 mcg tablets
    #C
    Take 1 tablet d

[ ] Contents are labeled
    unless checked

May be refilled 0 1 2 3 4

Signed _____ M.D.
Date _____ 19___ DEA No. _____

Figure C-8

App. C / Practice Prescriptions 161

H₂ blocker
Ulcers.
reduce amt
of HCl in
stomach.

```
PAT SMITH, M.D.
27 Oak Leaf Lane
Baltimore, MD  12121
Phone: 322-7890          Name_____
                         Address_____
                                    Age_____

Rx   Zantac 150 mg Tablets
        #100
        ÷ BID

[ ] Contents are labeled    May be refilled 0 1 2 3 4
    unless checked
                            Signed_____ M.D.
                            Date_____19___ DEA No._____
```

Figure C-9

Ulcers
H₂ blocker

```
PAT SMITH, M.D.
27 Oak Leaf Lane
Baltimore, MD  12121
Phone: 322-7890          Name_____
                         Address_____
                                    Age_____

Rx   Tagamet 300 mg/5ml
       Disp 480 ml
     Sig. 800 mg hs

[ ] Contents are labeled    May be refilled 0 1 2 3 4
    unless checked
                            Signed_____ M.D.
                            Date_____19___ DEA No._____
```

Figure C-10

3 teaspoon = 1 tablespoon.
1 tsp = 5 ml
1 tb = 15 ml

App. C / Practice Prescriptions

PAT SMITH, M.D.
27 Oak Leaf Lane
Baltimore, MD 12121
Phone: 322-7890

Name_____
Address_____
Age_____

Rx Xanax 0.5 mg Tabs.
      #30
    S. 0.5mg TID - no more than
       4 mg per day. No ETOH

[ ] Contents are labeled unless checked
May be refilled 0 1 2 3 4
Signed_____ M.D.
Date_____ 19___ DEA No._____

Margin note: Benzodiazepine anxiolytic tranquilizer

Figure C-11

PAT SMITH, M.D.
27 Oak Leaf Lane
Baltimore, MD 12121
Phone: 322-7890

Name_____
Address_____
Age_____

Rx Tabs. Coumadin 5mg
    (disp) d.t.d. 30
    S. 5mg daily - DO NOT TAKE ASA

[ ] Contents are labeled unless checked
May be refilled 0 1 2 3 4
Signed_____ M.D.
Date_____ 19___ DEA No._____

Margin note: Vasodilator (opens blood vessels) Calcium channel blocker ↓ BP - Anti angina anticoagulant

Figure C-12

App. C / Practice Prescriptions   163

Calcium channel blocker
Vasodilator (opens
blood vessels)

PAT SMITH, M.D.
27 Oak Leaf Lane
Baltimore, MD 12121
Phone: 322-7890

Name_____
Address_____
Age_____

℞ Cardizem 30 mg tablets
   120
   ī QID ac and hs

[ ] Contents are labeled unless checked

May be refilled 0 1 2 3 4

Signed_____ M.D.
Date_____ 19___ DEA No._____

Figure C-13

Pain killer

PAT SMITH, M.D.
27 Oak Leaf Lane
Baltimore, MD 12121
Phone: 322-7890

Name_____
Address_____
Age_____

℞ Darvocet-N 50 Tabs
   # XXX
   Si: ī q 4° prn pain

[ ] Contents are labeled unless checked

May be refilled 0 1 2 3 4

Signed_____ M.D.
Date_____ 19___ DEA No._____

Figure C-14

App. C / Practice Prescriptions

PAT SMITH, M.D.
27 Oak Leaf Lane
Baltimore, MD 12121
Phone: 322-7890

Name_____
Address_____
Age_____

Rx Valium 5mg
    Tabs # XX
S: ss̄ tab 3-4 x d. May have 1 tab
hs prn muscle spasms.
        NO ETOH

[ ] Contents are labeled   May be refilled 0 1 2 3 4
    unless checked
                            Signed_____M.D.
                            Date_____ 19___ DEA No._____

Margin note: Benzodiazepine tranquilizer ↓ libido

Figure C-15

PAT SMITH, M.D.
27 Oak Leaf Lane
Baltimore, MD 12121
Phone: 322-7890

Name_____
Address_____
Age_____

Rx Motrin 400mg Tabs
    #40
Sig: 400 mg to 800mg TID
     w/ food prn pain

[ ] Contents are labeled   May be refilled 0 1 2 3 4
    unless checked
                            Signed_____M.D.
                            Date_____ 19___ DEA No._____

Margin note: Pain killer

Figure C-16

App. C / Practice Prescriptions   165

PAT SMITH, M.D.
27 Oak Leaf Lane
Baltimore, MD 12121
Phone: 322-7890

Name_____

Address_____

Age_____

Rx Sumycin Caps 0.250 Gm
    #40

Sig: Open 1 cap in 1 oz. H_2O and
     rinse mouth QID

[ ] Contents are labeled   May be refilled 0 1 2 3 4
    unless checked
                              Signed_____ M.D.
                              Date_____ 19___ DEA No._____

Figure C-17

PAT SMITH, M.D.
27 Oak Leaf Lane
Baltimore, MD 12121
Phone: 322-7890

Name_____

Address_____

Age_____

Rx Theo-Dur tablets
    #100 X 300mg

S: 450mg Q12H for wheezing

[ ] Contents are labeled   May be refilled 0 1 2 3 4
    unless checked
                              Signed_____ M.D.
                              Date_____ 19___ DEA No._____

Figure C-18

166 App. C / Practice Prescriptions

PAT SMITH, M.D.
27 Oak Leaf Lane
Baltimore, MD 12121
Phone: 322-7890

Name_____
Address_____
Age_____

Rx Tabs Halcion 0.25 mg
XXX

Sig: Take i hs prn sleep

[ ] Contents are labeled unless checked

May be refilled 0 1 2 3 4

Signed_____ M.D.
Date_____ 19___ DEA No._____

Figure C-19

PAT SMITH, M.D.
27 Oak Leaf Lane
Baltimore, MD 12121
Phone: 322-7890

Name_____
Address_____
Age_____

Rx Dilantin 100mg Caps.
dtd #100

Sig: 400mg stat, 100mg BD 1st day, then 100mg TID thereafter.

[ ] Contents are labeled unless checked

May be refilled 0 1 2 3 4

Signed_____ M.D.
Date_____ 19___ DEA No._____

Figure C-20

App. C / Practice Prescriptions 167

PAT SMITH, M.D.
27 Oak Leaf Lane
Baltimore, MD 12121
Phone: 322-7890

Name_____
Address_____
                              Age_____

℞ Monistat Vaginal Cr. 2%
     45 Gm.
Sig: 1 applicatorful vaginally
     daily hs X 7d

[ ] Contents are labeled   May be refilled 0 1 2 3 4
    unless checked
                            Signed_____ M.D.
                            Date_____ 19___ DEA No._____

Figure C-21

PAT SMITH, M.D.
27 Oak Leaf Lane
Baltimore, MD 12121
Phone: 322-7890

Name_____
Address_____
                              Age_____

℞ Slow-K (8mEq.)
   # sixty
Sig: ii d. Swallow whole.

[ ] Contents are labeled   May be refilled 0 1 2 3 4
    unless checked
                            Signed_____ M.D.
                            Date_____ 19___ DEA No._____

Figure C-22

PAT SMITH, M.D.
27 Oak Leaf Lane
Baltimore, MD 12121
Phone: 322-7890

Name_____

Address_____

Age_____

℞ Caps. Feldene 20 mg.
#30
Sig. ī q d w/food or milk.

[ ] Contents are labeled unless checked

May be refilled 0 1 2 3 4

Signed_____M.D.

Date_____19___ DEA No._____

Figure C-23

PAT SMITH, M.D.
27 Oak Leaf Lane
Baltimore, MD 12121
Phone: 322-7890

Name_____

Address_____

Age_____

℞ Ortho-Novum 2mg
d. ī pack
ī tab daily days 5-25 of
menstrual cycle.

[ ] Contents are labeled unless checked

May be refilled 0 1 2 3 4

Signed_____M.D.

Date_____19___ DEA No._____

Figure C-24

App. C / Practice Prescriptions 169

Taken out of market

PAT SMITH, M.D.
27 Oak Leaf Lane
Baltimore, MD 12121
Phone: 322-7890

Name_____
Address_____
Age_____

R̲x Nicorette 2mg gum
Disp. ī box of 96
Sig: ut dict per instructions. No more than 30 pieces per day.

[ ] Contents are labeled unless checked   May be refilled 0 1 2 3 4

Signed_____ M.D.
Date_____ 19___ DEA No._____

Figure C-25

PAT SMITH, M.D.
27 Oak Leaf Lane
Baltimore, MD 12121
Phone: 322-7890

Name_____
Address_____
Age_____

R̲x Compazine 25mg Suppos.
XII
S: ī PR BID for N/V

[ ] Contents are labeled unless checked   May be refilled 0 1 2 3 4

Signed_____ M.D.
Date_____ 19___ DEA No._____

Figure C-26

ANSWERS

Figure C-1

Generic name: clotrimazole
Trade name: Lotrimin
Strength: 1%
Dosage form: cream
Amount dispensed: 15 grams
Directions to the patient: Apply to affected area twice a day in the morning and evening.

Figure C-2

Generic name: nitroglycerin
Trade name: Transderm-Nitro
Strength: 2.5 mg.
Dosage form: patch
Amount dispensed: 30
Directions to the patient: Apply 1 patch every 24 hours.

Figure C-3

Generic name: timolol
Trade name: Timoptic
Strength: 0.25%
Dosage form: ophthalmic drops
Amount dispensed: 1 bottle
Directions to the patient: Instill 1 drop to both eyes twice a day.

Figure C-4

Generic name: metaproterenol
Trade name: Alupent
Strength: 225 mg. per inhaler
Dosage form: inhalant
Amount dispensed: one inhaler unit
Directions to the patient: Inhale 2 puffs every 3 to 4 hours. Use no more than 12 puffs per day.

Figure C-5

Generic name: gemfibrozil
Trade name: Lopid
Strength: 300 mg.
Dosage form: capsule (oral)
Amount dispensed: 100
Directions to the patient: Take 2 capsules $\frac{1}{2}$ hour before breakfast and 2 capsules $\frac{1}{2}$ hour before dinner.

Figure C-6

Generic name: conjugated estrogens
Trade name: Premarin
Strength: 1.25 mg.
Dosage form: tablet (oral)
Amount dispensed: 40
Directions to the patient: Take 1 tablet in the morning and evening for 20 days, rest 10 days, and resume schedule.
(*Note*: This drug is to be dispensed with a patient package insert—PPI.)

Figure C-7

Generic name: propranolol
Trade name: Inderal
Strength: 40 mg.
Dosage form: tablet (oral)
Amount dispensed: 50
Directions to the patient: Take 2 tablets daily (1 tablet in the morning and 1 tablet in the evening).

Figure C-8

Generic name: levothyroxine
Trade name: Synthroid
Strength: 100 micrograms (or 0.1 mg.)
Dosage form: tablet (oral)
Amount dispensed: 100
Directions to the patient: Take 1 tablet daily.

Figure C-9

Generic name: ranitidine
Trade name: Zantac
Strength: 150 mg.
Dosage form: tablet (oral)
Amount dispensed: 100
Directions to the patient: Take 1 tablet twice a day.

Figure C-10

Generic name: cimetidine
Trade name: Tagamet
Strength: 300 mg. per teaspoonful
Dosage form: liquid (oral)
Amount dispensed: 480 ml. or 1 pint
Directions to the patient: Take $2\frac{1}{2}$ teaspoonful at bedtime.
(*Note*: Actual calculations indicate 2.6 teaspoonsful at bedtime. However, patients understand $2\frac{1}{2}$ teaspoonsful, which measure within an accurate dosage.)

Figure C-11

Generic name: alprazolam
Trade name: Xanax
Strength: 0.5 mg.
Dosage form: tablet (oral)
Amount dispensed: 30
Directions to the patient: Take 1 tablet 3 times a day. Do NOT take more than 8 tablets per day. NO ALCOHOL.

Figure C-12

Generic name: warfarin
Trade name: Coumadin
Strength: 5 mg.
Dosage form: tablet (oral)
Amount dispensed: 30
Directions to the patient: Take 1 tablet daily. DO NOT TAKE ASPIRIN.

Figure C-13

Generic name: diltiazem
Trade name: Cardizem
Strength: 30 mg.
Dosage form: tablet (oral)
Amount dispensed: 120
Directions to the patient: Take 1 tablet 4 times a day before meals and at bedtime.

Figure C-14

Generic name: propoxyphene/acetaminophen
Trade name: Darvocet-N
Strength: propoxyphene 50 mg./acetaminophen 325 mg.
Dosage form: tablet (oral)
Amount dispensed: 30
Directions to the patient: Take 1 tablet every 4 hours as needed for pain.

Figure C-15

Generic name: diazepam
Trade name: Valium
Strength: 5 mg.
Dosage form: tablet (oral)
Amount dispensed: 20
Directions to the patient: Take $\frac{1}{2}$ tablet 3 or 4 times a day. May have 1 tablet at bedtime as needed for muscle spasms. NO ALCOHOL.

Figure C-16

Generic name: ibuprofen
Trade name: Motrin (or Rufen)
Strength: 400 mg.
Dosage form: tablet (oral)
Amount dispensed: 40
Directions to the patient: Take 1 or 2 tablets 3 times a day with food as needed for pain.

Figure C-17

Generic name: tetracycline
Trade name: Sumycin (or Achromycin V)
Strength: 250 mg.
Dosage form: capsule (oral)
Amount dispensed: 40
Directions to the patient: Open 1 capsule in 1 ounce of water and rinse mouth 4 times a day.

Figure C-18

Generic name: theophylline
Trade name: Theo-Dur (or Slo-Bid, Slo-Phyllin)
Strength: 300 mg.
Dosage form: tablet (oral)
Amount dispensed: 100
Directions to the patient: Take $1\frac{1}{2}$ tablets every 12 hours for wheezing.

Figure C-19

Generic name: triazolam
Trade name: Halcion
Strength: 0.25 mg.
Dosage form: tablet (oral)
Amount dispensed: 30
Directions to the patient: Take 1 tablet at bedtime as needed for sleep.

Figure C-20

Generic name: phenytoin
Trade name: Dilantin
Strength: 100 mg.
Dosage form: capsule (oral)
Amount dispensed: 100
Directions to the patient: Take 4 capsules at once, 1 capsule twice a day for the first day, then 1 capsule 3 times a day thereafter.

Figure C-21

Generic name: miconazole
Trade name: Monistat
Strength: 2%
Dosage form: vaginal cream
Amount dispensed: 45 grams
Directions to the patient: Insert 1 applicatorful vaginally daily at bedtime for 7 days.

Figure C-22

Generic name: potassium
Trade name: Slow-K (or Micro-K, K-Tab, Klotrix, K-Lyte, Kaon) (*Note*: Strengths vary for each product)
Strength: 8 milliequivalents
Dosage form: tablet (oral)
Amount dispensed: 60
Directions to the patient: Take 2 tablets daily. SWALLOW WHOLE.

Figure C-23

Generic name: piroxicam
Trade name: Feldene
Strength: 20 mg.
Dosage form: capsule (oral)
Amount dispensed: 30
Directions to the patient: Take 1 capsule every day with food or milk.

Figure C-24

Generic name: norethindrone/mestranol
Trade name: Ortho-Novum
Strength: norethindrone 2 mg./mestranol 0.10 mg.
Dosage form: tablet (oral)
Amount dispensed: 1 pack (contains 21 tablets)
Directions to the patient: Take 1 tablet daily, days 5–25 of the menstrual cycle.

Figure C-25

Generic name: nicotine
Trade name: Nicorette
Strength: 2 mg.
Dosage form: gum (oral)
Amount dispensed: 96
Directions to the patient: Chew as directed per instructions. Chew no more than 30 pieces per day.

Figure C-26

Generic name: prochlorperazine
Trade name: Compazine
Strength: 25 mg.
Dosage form: suppository (rectal)
Amount dispensed: 12
Directions to the patient: Insert 1 suppository rectally twice a day for nausea and vomiting.

APPENDIX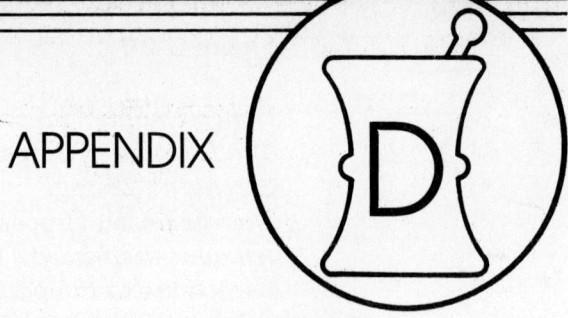

Practice Hospital Orders

The Physician's Order Record is the primary method used to communicate a hospitalized patient's medication needs to the pharmacy. Therefore, you must be able to review the order and highlight the information needed by pharmacy staff to complete the physician's request for drugs. This appendix contains actual hospital orders that have been rewritten with special highlights (lettered arrows) added to emphasize practice with phrases, abbreviations, and special terminology.

Read each practice hospital order (Physician's Order Record) entirely. Note the items highlighted by lettered arrows. Interpret each of these highlighted items. Answers follow the practice orders.

App. D / Practice Hospital Orders 177

PATIENT:	MEMORIAL HOSPITAL
AGE:	BALTIMORE, MARYLAND
SEX:	PHYSICIAN'S ORDER RECORD
RACE:	
CHART NO.	BEAR DOWN ON HARD SURFACE WITH BALL POINT PEN

GENERIC EQUIVALENT IS AUTHORIZED UNLESS CHECKED IN THIS COLUMN

ALLERGY OR SENSITIVITY: none
DIAGNOSIS: S/P (R) wrist Fx ← A
COMPLETED OR DISCONTINUED

DATE	TIME	ORDERS	PHYSICIAN'S SIG.	NAME	DATE	TIME
6/22	6:15A	Admit to Med C				
		Condition: stable				
		diet 4 Gm Na+ ↓ salt diet				
		activity - bedrest				
		vital Q4°				
		Med:				
		Capoten 12.5 mg P.O. BID ← B				
		C → Colace 100mg P.O. QD				
		D → HCTZ 50mg PO QD				
		E → Clonidine - 1 patch 1 a week				
		F → Tylenol with Codeine (#3) PO Q4-6° prn				
		G → Heparin SQ 5000u q12°				
		IVF D5 ½ NS KVO ← H				
		Schedule ① Holter ② Cat Scan				
		for AM ③ EEG ④ Echo				
		— MD				
6/23	9A	Prepare for OR				
		NPO				
		I → Scrub wrist c̄ povidone-iodine scrub				
		Diazepam 10 mg IV ← J				
		— MD				

PHARMACY COPY

Figure D-1

App. D / Practice Hospital Orders

MEMORIAL HOSPITAL
BALTIMORE, MARYLAND
PHYSICIAN'S ORDER RECORD

BEAR DOWN ON HARD SURFACE WITH BALL POINT PEN

PATIENT:
AGE:
SEX:
RACE:
CHART NO.

GENERIC EQUIVALENT IS AUTHORIZED UNLESS CHECKED IN THIS COLUMN ✓

ALLERGY OR SENSITIVITY TO: NKA
NONE KNOWN ☐ SIGNED:

DIAGNOSIS: ASHD

COMPLETED OR DISCONTINUED

DATE	TIME	ORDERS	PHYSICIAN'S SIG.	NAME	DATE	TIME
2/7	3p	TNG s.l. 1/150 gr. ī Now (under tongue) — may repeat Q5' × 3 doses ← A				
		B → Maalox 30cc alternate c̄ AMPHOGEL 30cc Q2° w.a.				
		Isosorbide L.A. 40 MG. P.O. Q8° ← C				
		D → Verapamil s.r. 240 mg. ½ tab QD (P.O.)				
		Zantac 150 MG P.O. Q12H ← E				
		F → Lubriderm at bedside PRN USE				
		(Tylenol) APAP ī tabs. P.O. Q4° PRN HA (or ī SUPPOS (650 mg)) ← G				12 table
		H → Halcion 0.25 mg PO QHS PRN				
		Baby ASA ī P.O. QD ← I				
		lactulose 15 cc PO QD ← J				
		Dietary Consult in AM.				
			MD			

PHARMACY COPY

Figure D-2

App. D / Practice Hospital Orders 179

MEMORIAL HOSPITAL
BALTIMORE, MARYLAND
PHYSICIAN'S ORDER RECORD

BEAR DOWN ON HARD SURFACE WITH BALL POINT PEN

PATIENT:
AGE:
SEX:
RACE:
CHART NO.

GENERIC EQUIVALENT IS AUTHORIZED UNLESS CHECKED IN THIS COLUMN

ALLERGY OR SENSITIVITY TO: diflunisal, ibuprofen, PCN
DIAGNOSIS: UGI bleeding ← A
NONE KNOWN ☐ SIGNED: [signature]
COMPLETED OR DISCONTINUED

DATE	TIME	ORDERS	PHYSICIAN'S SIG.	NAME	DATE	TIME
7/2	1645	Admit to MED A DRs P/C/N				
		Condition: fair				
		Vitals: Q4°×3, then Q shift.				
		Act: Bedrest tonight, then ad lib				
		I and O please				
		Diet: CLD tonite ← C				
		NPO p̄ MN				
		Schedule upper endoscopy in AM.				
		Meds —				
		E → Maalox 30 cc PO q4° ← D				
		Zantac 50 mg IV q8° (3 IV bags)				
		Folic acid 1 mg PO QD ← F				
		G → KCl 20 mEq in OJ QD × 2 days				
		Labs: Stat CBC tonite p̄ 1 unit PRBCs				
		AM Labs: CBC, SMA 7, PT, PTT				
		Call H.O. Systolic BP <100, >180				
		HR <60, >100				
		H → IVF ½ NS @ 100cc/hr × 3L				
		I → O₂ NC 2L				
		Vit K 10 mg IM QD × 3d				
		↗ ies coagulate	[signature] MD			

PHARMACY COPY

Figure D-3

App. D / Practice Hospital Orders

MEMORIAL HOSPITAL
BALTIMORE, MARYLAND
PHYSICIAN'S ORDER RECORD

PATIENT:
AGE:
SEX:
RACE:
CHART NO.

BEAR DOWN ON HARD SURFACE WITH BALL POINT PEN

GENERIC EQUIVALENT IS AUTHORIZED UNLESS CHECKED IN THIS COLUMN

ALLERGY OR SENSITIVITY TO __∅__
NONE KNOWN ☐ SIGNED: _m_

DIAGNOSIS: UTI

COMPLETED OR DISCONTINUED

DATE	TIME	ORDERS	PHYSICIAN'S SIG.	NAME	DATE	TIME
7/15	8A	Admit to Dr. ___ / Urology				
		S/P ® ureteral stone extraction				
		Cond: stable				
		Vitals: Per routine				
		Act: Bedrest				
		Diet: CLD				
		A→ IVF: D5 ½ NS c̄ 20 mEq KCl @ 100 ml/H 10 hrs 10⁹ ×1 / 1000				
		Meds: 1000ml in bag so				
		AMPICILLIN 500mg IV Q6° ←B				
		C→ GENT 80 mg IV Q8°				
		Percocet ī - īī PO Q 4° PRN ←D 12 tabs				
		E→ (-OR- DEMEROL 50mg c̄ VISTARIL 50mg IM Q4° PRN)				
		diuretic to remove stone				
		Lasix 20mg IV now ←F				
		Labs: CBC c. diff				
		_m_ MD				
		for BP ← CAPTOPRIL 25 mg PO BID ←G				
		HCTZ 25 mg PO QAM				
		H→ Trental 400 mg PO BID ←I				
		Halcion 0.25 mg PO @ HS PRN				
		J↑ _m_ MD				

PHARMACY COPY

Figure D-4

App. D / Practice Hospital Orders 181

MEMORIAL HOSPITAL
BALTIMORE, MARYLAND
PHYSICIAN'S ORDER RECORD

BEAR DOWN ON HARD SURFACE WITH BALL POINT PEN

PATIENT:
AGE:
SEX:
RACE:
CHART NO.

GENERIC EQUIVALENT IS AUTHORIZED UNLESS CHECKED IN THIS COLUMN

ALLERGY OR SENSITIVITY TO: Ragweed, fish
DIAGNOSIS: Pneumonia
COMPLETED OR DISCONTINUED

DATE	TIME	ORDERS	PHYSICIAN'S SIG.	NAME	DATE	TIME
6/14	10³⁰ᵖ	Admit to Med A				
		Cond. Fair				
		Vitals - Q shift				
		Act: UP AD LIB ← A				
		Diet: Regular				
		B → IVF: D5 ½ NS c̄ 10 mEq/L. @ 50 cc/L. × 3L			60 hrs 50/1000 × 3	
		Meds:				
		C → Cefuroxime 0.75 gm. IV Q8° — 1ST dose STAT				
		bronchodilator E Alupent inhaler ÏÏ puffs Q6° ← 8 puffs D				
		Tonite: ABG ← E				
6/15	8¹⁵A	40 mEq KCl RTS ← F				
		G → 10 mEq KCl in 100 cc NS × 4 runs over 1° ea.				
		portable CXR in AM				
		H → Temp PR. APAP ÏÏ (650 mg) T > 101⁵				
6/16	1 AM	Halcion 0.125 mg. PO now ← I				
		V.O. Dr.				
6/17	7A	Start gent. 55 mg Q 8 H				
		↑ injection				
		J				

PHARMACY COPY

Figure D-5

MEMORIAL HOSPITAL
BALTIMORE, MARYLAND
PHYSICIAN'S ORDER RECORD

PATIENT:
AGE:
SEX:
RACE:
CHART NO.

BEAR DOWN ON HARD SURFACE WITH BALL POINT PEN

✓ GENERIC EQUIVALENT IS AUTHORIZED UNLESS CHECKED IN THIS COLUMN

ALLERGY OR SENSITIVITY TO: NKDA ← A
NONE KNOWN ☐ SIGNED: Sm

DIAGNOSIS: ASCVD ← B

DATE	TIME	ORDERS	PHYSICIAN'S SIG.
7/5		Admit to 10th Floor	
		Cond. Fair	
		VS: Q4H x 24H then Q shift	
		Act: OOB c̄ Assistance ← C	
		Diet: 4 Gm Na+ diet	
		EKG QAM x 3D	
		O₂ 2L/min. via NC ← D	
		Meds:	
		F → Digox 0.25 mg. po. qam ← E	
		Kondremul 15cc po qhs on M.W.F	
		Tylenol ii Q4H PRN ← G	
		H → Xanax 0.25 mg qhs prn P.O. ← I	
		Dig. level in am	
			Sm MD
		J → D/C Xanax. give flurazepam 15 mg	
		qhs prn. V.O. Sm	

PHARMACY COPY

Figure D-6

App. D / Practice Hospital Orders   183

PATIENT: AGE: SEX: RACE: CHART NO.	MEMORIAL HOSPITAL BALTIMORE, MARYLAND PHYSICIAN'S ORDER RECORD

BEAR DOWN ON HARD SURFACE WITH BALL POINT PEN

GENERIC EQUIVALENT IS AUTHORIZED UNLESS CHECKED IN THIS COLUMN

ALLERGY OR SENSITIVITY: ASA ← A
NONE KNOWN ☐ SIGNED:

DIAGNOSIS: chest pain
CHF ← B

COMPLETED OR DISCONTINUED

DATE	TIME	ORDERS	PHYSICIAN'S SIG.	NAME	DATE	TIME
1/14	715	Admit to Telemetry				
		Cond: Fair				
		Activity: Bedrest				
		Diet: NPO except Meds				
		VS q4h				
		Meds:				
		① Dig. 0.25mg IV q6° × 2 doses ← C				
		then Dig. 0.25mg PO QAM				
D→		② Demerol 25mg IM c̄ Hydroxyzine 25mg IM				
		q6H prn				
E→		③ Heparin SQ 5000u Q12H				
F→		④ Thiamine 100mg IM Tonite and QD×3D				
G→		⑤ MgSO4 1gm IM to each buttocks				
H→		IVF: D5NS c̄ 30 mEq KCl at 250cc/hr. × 2L.				
		then ↓ rate to 125cc per h				
		add ½ amp MVI ⎫ to bottle #2 ← I				
		add 1 mg folate ⎭				
		Labs: SMA-7, amylase in AM				
		Dig. Level in AM				
		Echocardiogram				
		EKG QAM × 3d ← J				
		Glenn, MD				

PHARMACY COPY

Figure D-7

App. D / Practice Hospital Orders

MEMORIAL HOSPITAL
BALTIMORE, MARYLAND
PHYSICIAN'S ORDER RECORD

PATIENT:
AGE:
SEX:
RACE:
CHART NO.

BEAR DOWN ON HARD SURFACE WITH BALL POINT PEN

GENERIC EQUIVALENT IS AUTHORIZED UNLESS CHECKED IN THIS COLUMN

ALLERGY OR SENSITIVITY TO: PCN ← A
NONE KNOWN ☐ SIGNED:

DIAGNOSIS: Acute exacerbation of COPD, Bronchitis

COMPLETED OR DISCONTINUED

DATE	TIME	ORDERS	PHYSICIAN'S SIG.	NAME	DATE	TIME
7/9	8AM	Admit to Med C				
		Cond – guarded				
		VS per floor routine				
		Activities as tolerated				
		Diet: 1800 Kcal ADA, 4g Na				
		Meds:				
		Aminophylline 500mg. in 500cc NS at 40cc/hr. ← C				
		B → Lasix 40 mg po BID				
		D → nitroglycerin patch 10 cm² QD				
		E → tolazamide 250 mg po QD				
		F → Slow-K ii 9 AM				
		G → alupent nebulizers 0.3cc/3cc NS q4°				
		H → ampicillin 250 mg po TID				
		Labs:				
		Aminophylline level tonight and in AM				
		J → Call H.O. for T > 100.5				
		Systolic BP > 200				
		Diastolic BP < 60				
		(signature) MD				

PHARMACY COPY

Figure D-8

App. D / Practice Hospital Orders

MEMORIAL HOSPITAL
BALTIMORE, MARYLAND
PHYSICIAN'S ORDER RECORD

BEAR DOWN ON HARD SURFACE WITH BALL POINT PEN

GENERIC EQUIVALENT IS AUTHORIZED UNLESS CHECKED IN THIS COLUMN

ALLERGY OR SENSITIVITY TO: Codeine, Darvocet-N
DIAGNOSIS: Syncope

DATE	TIME	ORDERS
12/3	1p	① Admit to Med A
		② Cond - stable
		③ Diet - CL diet × 2d
		④ ACT - OOB ad lib
		⑤ Vitals - q 4° × 2×, then per routine
		⑥ MEDS:
		→ phenytoin 100mg q8° ← A
		B → KCl 25 mEq po now, then qd.
		Thiamine 100mg po qd ← C
		D → folic acid 1mg q A.M.
		MVI 1 po qd ← E
		F → ⑦ IVF - D5·NS @ 75cc/hr × 2L
		G → ⑧ V.O. MD -
		H → 1g mg SO₄ each buttock × 1
		I → triazolam 0.125mg qhs prn sleep
		⑨ AM Labs - CBC, SMA, phenytoin level
		⑩ EKG, EEG in AM
		J → ⑪ Call H/O if SOB or seizing
		—— , MD

PHARMACY COPY

Figure D-9

App. D / Practice Hospital Orders

MEMORIAL HOSPITAL
BALTIMORE, MARYLAND
PHYSICIAN'S ORDER RECORD

PATIENT:
AGE:
SEX:
RACE:
CHART NO.

BEAR DOWN ON HARD SURFACE WITH BALL POINT PEN

GENERIC EQUIVALENT IS AUTHORIZED UNLESS CHECKED IN THIS COLUMN

ALLERGY OR SENSITIVITY TO: ∅ ← A
NONE KNOWN ☐ SIGNED: ___

DIAGNOSIS: S/P hernia repair

COMPLETED OR DISCONTINUED

DATE	TIME	ORDERS	PHYSICIAN'S SIG.	NAME	DATE	TIME
1/8	4pm	Post Op Orders				

Admit to RR
Condition – stable
VS: q4° x 2, then q shift ← B
Diet: Regular

D5 ½ NS W/ 20 mEq KCl/L ← C
run @ 100 cc/hr
D/C when taking PO well ← D
Meds:
E → Meperidine 50mg IM q3°h prn pain
F → Vistaril 25 mg IM q3H prn pain
G → Halcion 0.25 mg PO q hs prn
H → LOC prn
Lance foot sore in AM
I → cefazolin 1 Gm IV in RR

J → Call H.O. T > 101.5
BP > 180/100 or
< 80/60

Sm, MD

PHARMACY COPY

Figure D-10

ANSWERS

Figure D-1

A. Diagnosis-condition: fracture of the right wrist.
B. Capoten, 12.5 mg. orally twice a day.
C. Colace, 100 mg. orally every day.
D. Hydrochlorothiazide, 50 mg. orally every day.
E. Clonidine-1 patch, one patch per week.
F. Tylenol with codeine (#3 refers to 30 mg. of codeine in this product), one tablet orally every 4 to 6 hours as needed.
G. Heparin, 5000 units every 12 hours subcutaneously.
H. Intravenous fluids, dextrose 5 percent in $\frac{1}{2}$ normal saline, keep vein open.
I. Scrub wrist with povidone-iodine scrub.
J. Diazepam, 10 mg. intravenously.

Figure D-2

A. Nitroglycerin sublingual $\frac{1}{150}$ grain, one now and may repeat every 5 minutes for 3 doses.
B. Maalox 30 cc., alternate with Amphogel 30 cc. every 2 hours while awake.
C. Isosorbide long acting 40 mg., one orally every 8 hours.
D. Verapamil sustained release 240 mg., $\frac{1}{2}$ tablet every day (orally).
E. Zantac, 150 mg. orally every 12 hours.
F. Lubriderm at bedside, use as needed.
G. Acetaminophen, 2 tablets orally every 4 hours as needed for headache [or 1 suppository (strength = 650 mg.)].
H. Halcion, 0.25 mg. orally every bedtime if needed.
I. Baby aspirin, one tablet orally every day.
J. Lactulose, 15 cc.(1 tablespoonful) orally every day.

Figure D-3

A. Diagnosis: upper gastrointestinal bleeding.
B. Allergy or sensitivity: ibuprofen, diflunisal, penicillin.
C. Diet: clear liquid diet tonight, nothing by mouth after midnight.
D. Maalox, 30 cc. orally every 4 hours.
E. Zantac, 50 mg. intravenously every 8 hours.
F. Folic acid, 1 mg. orally every day.
G. Potassium chloride, 20 milliequivalents in orange juice every day for 2 days.
H. Call house officer if systolic blood pressure is less than 100 or greater than 180, heart rate less than 60 or greater than 100.

I. Intravenous fluids, ½ normal saline to run at 100 cc. per hour for 3 liters.

J. Vitamin K, 10 mg. intramuscularly every day for 3 days.

Figure D-4

A. Intravenous fluids: dextrose 5 percent in ½ normal saline with 20 milliequivalents of potassium chloride to run at 100 milliliters per hour.

B. Ampicillin, 500 mg. intravenously every 6 hours.

C. Gentamicin, 80 mg. intravenously every 8 hours.

D. Percocet, one or 2 tablets orally every 4 hours as needed.

E. (or Demerol 50 mg. and Vistaril 50 mg. intramuscularly every 4 hours as needed).

F. Lasix, 20 mg. intravenously now.

G. Captopril, 25 mg. orally twice a day.

H. Hydrochlorothiazide, 25 mg. orally every morning.

I. Trental, 400 mg. orally twice a day.

J. Halcion, 0.25 mg. orally every bedtime as needed.

Figure D-5

A. Activities: up as desired.

B. Intravenous fluids: dextrose 5 percent in ½ normal saline with 10 milliequivalents per liter for 3 liters. (*Note:* The order does not specify the drug to be used that will supply 10 mEq. You know the drug must be potassium chloride. However, you DO NOT assume the physician wants potassium chloride. Call the physician and be sure to secure a Physician's Order rewritten by the physician for the appropriate drug order.)

C. Cefuroxime, 0.75 Gm. intravenously every 8 hours. The first dose is to be given immediately.

D. Alupent inhaler, 2 puffs every 6 hours.

E. Tonight: arterial blood gases.

F. 40 milliequivalents of potassium chloride is to be returned to stock.

G. 10 milliequivalents of potassium chloride in 100 cc. of normal saline for 4 runs, each to run for 1 hour.

H. Take temperature rectally. Acetaminophen, 2 tablets (650 mg. total strength) for temperature greater than 101.5 degrees.

I. Halcion, 0.125 mg. orally now. Verbal order by physician.

J. Start gentamicin, 55 mg. every 8 hours.

Figure D-6

A. Allergy or sensitivity: no known drug allergies.

B. Diagnosis: arteriosclerotic cardiovascular disease.

C. Activities: out of bed with assistance.
D. Oxygen, 2 liters per minute via nasal cannula.
E. Digoxin, 0.25 mg. orally every morning.
F. Kondremul, 15 cc. (1 tablespoonful) orally every bedtime on Monday, Wednesday, and Friday.
G. Tylenol, 2 tablets every 4 hours as needed.
H. Digoxin level in the morning.
I. Xanax, 0.25 mg. every bedtime as needed. Orally.
J. Discontinue Xanax. Give flurazepam 15 mg. every bedtime as needed. Verbal order by physician.

Figure D-7

A. Allergy or sensitivity: aspirin.
B. Diagnosis: chest pain, congestive heart failure.
C. Digoxin, 0.25 mg. intravenously every 6 hours for 2 doses, then digoxin, 0.25 mg. orally every morning.
D. Demerol, 25 mg. intramuscularly with hydroxyzine, 25 mg. intramuscularly every 6 hours as needed.
E. Heparin, 5000 units subcutaneously every 12 hours.
F. Thiamine, 100 mg. intramuscularly tonight and every day for 3 days.
G. Magnesium sulfate, 1 gram intramuscularly into each buttock.
H. Intravenous fluids: dextrose 5 percent in normal saline (normal saline = 0.9% sodium chloride solution) with 30 milliequivalents of potassium chloride to run at 250 cc. per hour for 2 liters, then decrease rate to 125 cc. per hour.
I. Add 1 ampoule of multivitamin infusion and 1 mg. of folic acid to bottle number 2 (that is, the 2nd liter bottle).
J. Perform an electrocardiogram every morning for 3 days.

Figure D-8

A. Allergy or sensitivity: penicillin.
B. Lasix, 40 mg. orally twice a day.
C. Aminophylline, 500 mg. in 500 cc. of normal saline to run at 40 cc. per hour.
D. Nitroglycerin patch, 10 square centimeters, apply one every day.
E. Tolazamide, 250 mg. orally every day.
F. Slow-K, 2 tablets every morning.
G. Alupent nebulizers, 0.3 cc. per 3 cc. of normal saline every 4 hours.
H. Ampicillin, 250 mg. orally 3 times a day.
I. Laboratory to do an aminophylline blood level tonight and in the morning.
J. Call the house officer for temperature greater than 100.5 degrees,

systolic blood pressure greater than 200, or diastolic blood pressure less than 60.

Figure D-9

A. Phenytoin, 100 mg. every 8 hours.
B. Potassium chloride, 25 milliequivalents orally now, then every day.
C. Thiamine, 100 mg. orally every day.
D. Folic acid, 1 mg. every morning.
E. Multiple vitamin, one orally every day. (The oral indication, p.o., indicates that the vitamin is not an infusion.)
F. Intravenous fluids: dextrose 5 percent in normal saline to run at 75 cc. per hour for 2 liters.
G. Verbal order by physician.
H. 1 gram of magnesium sulfate in each buttock one time.
I. Triazolam, 0.125 mg. every bedtime as needed for sleep.
J. Call the house officer if the patient has shortness of breath or seizing.

Figure D-10

A. Allergy or sensitivity: none.
B. Vital signs: every 4 hours for 2 times, then every shift.
C. Dextrose 5 percent in $\frac{1}{2}$ normal saline with 20 milliequivalents of potassium chloride per liter to run at 100 cc. per hour.
D. Discontinue the intravenous fluids when the patient is able to take drugs, food, and liquids by mouth well.
E. Meperidine, 50 mg. intramuscularly every 3 hours as needed for pain.
F. Vistaril, 25 mg. intramuscularly every 3 hours as needed for pain.
G. Halcion, 0.25 mg. orally every bedtime as needed.
H. Laxative of choice as needed.
I. Cefazolin, 1 gram intravenously in the recovery room.
J. Call the house officer if the temperature is greater than 101.5 degrees, the blood pressure is greater than $\frac{180}{100}$ or less than $\frac{80}{60}$.

APPENDIX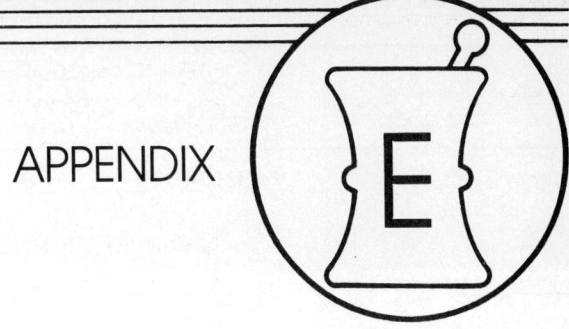

Common Laboratory Tests

Test	Abbreviation	Stools or Blood (B) or Urine (U)	Normal Range[a]	Abnormal Measurement Disorder Indicator
blood clotting tests		B		liver function, hemophilia, intestinal malabsorption, blood clotting disorders
prothrombin time	PT		10.5–12.5 seconds	
partial thromboplastin time	PTT		29–36 seconds	
bleeding time			less than 5 minutes	
complete blood count	CBC	B		anemia, infection
hematocrit	Hct		adult men: 42%–52% adult women: 37%–47% children: 31%–41% newborns: 44%–64%	
hemoglobin	Hb, Hgb		adult men: 14–18 Gm./dl. adult women: 12–16 Gm./dl. children: 10–15 Gm./dl. newborns: 14–25 Gm./dl.	
red blood cell count	RBC		adult men: 4.5–6.3 million per mm.³ adult women: 4.2–5.4 million per mm.³ children: 3.8–5.2 million per mm.³ newborns: 4.1–6.1 million per mm.³	
white blood cell count	WBC		4,000–10,000 per mm.³	
platelet count			150,000–350,000 per mm.³	

Test	Abbreviation	Stools or Blood (B) or Urine (U)	Normal Range[a]	Abnormal Measurement Disorder Indicator
electrolyte tests	lytes	B		kidney disorders, improper body water balance, improper blood acidity
sodium	Na		134–145 mEq./L.	
potassium	K		3.5–5.5 mEq./L.	
chloride	Cl		96–110 mEq./L.	
bicarbonate	HCO_3		24–30 mEq./L.	
erythrocyte sedimentation rate	ESR, sed rate	B	men: 0–10 mm. in 1 hour women: 0–20 mm. in 1 hour	inflammation, infection, cancer, rheumatoid arthritis
glucose tests		B		diabetes
glucose tolerance test	gtt		70–110 mg./dl.	
heart enzyme tests		B		heart attack
creatinine phosphokinase	CPK, Ck		0–180 IU/L.	
serum glutamic-oxalo-acetic transaminase	SGOT		1–50 IU/L.	
lactic dehydrogenase	LDH		90–250 IU/L.	
kidney function tests		B		kidney disorders
blood urea nitrogen	BUN		10–20 mg./dl.	
creatinine[b]	creat		0.5–1.5 mg./dl.	
creatinine clearance	CP		80–120 ml./minute	
lipid tests		B		predisposition to heart disease
cholesterol[c]			less than 190 mg. per dl. (under age 40) not more than 250 mg./dl. (over age 40)	
triglycerides			50–200 mg./dl.	
high density lipoproteins[d]	HDL		36–59 mg./dl.	
low density lipoproteins	LDL		70–180 mg./dl.	
liver function tests	LFT	B		liver dysfunction (jaundice, hepatitis, cancer, gallstones), digestive disorders, metabolism disorders, bone disorder, erythrocyte disorders
serum glutamic-oxalo-acetic transaminase	SGOT		1–50 IU/L.	
serum glutamic-pyruvic transaminase	SGPT		1–70 IU/L.	
lactic dehydrogenase	LDH		90–250 IU/L.	
alkaline phosphatase			0–70 u/L.	
bilirubin	bili		0.1–1.0 mg./dl.	
occult blood test		stools	absence	gastrointestinal (GI) disease, ulcerative collitis, polyps,

App. E / Common Laboratory Tests

Test	Abbreviation	Stools or Blood (B) or Urine (U)	Normal Range[a]	Abnormal Measurement Disorder Indicator
occult blood test (Continued)				hemorrhoids, fissures, cancer
routine urinalysis	UA	U		screen for kidney dysfunction, kidney stones, bladder stones, urinary tract infection, diabetes, hepatitis, liver disease, gallbladder disease, sickle cell anemia, gout (24-hour urine collection), leukemia (24-hour urine collection)
microscopic examination			negative findings	
culture			negative findings	
chemical examination[e]				
glucose			negative	
ketones			negative	
bilirubin			negative	
protein			negative	
urobilinogen			negative	
acidity	pH		approximately 7.0	
specific gravity	sp.gr.		1.006–1.030	
thyroid function tests		B		thyroid dysfunction
thyroxine	T_4		4.5–12.5 mcg./dl.	
tri-iodothyronine	T_3		23%–24%	
thyroid-stimulating hormone	TSH		less than 11 micro IU/ml.	
uric acid test		B	2.5–8.5 mg./dl.	gout, kidney failure, leukemia, cancer

[a] Normal range of values may vary according to the reference being used.
[b] Measurements vary with the size of the patient being tested.
[c] Measurements vary with the age of the patient being tested.
[d] Lower measurements indicate an increased risk of heart disease while higher measurements are associated with a decreased risk of heart disease.
[e] Specific substances are measured using a 24-hour urine collection:

calcium (Ca)	50–250 mg./24 hours	
protein	less than 50 mg./24 hours	
uric acid	250–750 mg./24 hours	
hormones		
vanillylmandelic acid (VMA)	less than 1–8 mg./24 hours	indicates pheochromocytoma, adrenal gland tumor
estrogen steroids		
17-ketosteroids (17-KS)	females: 5–15 mg./24 hours males: 5–23 mg./24 hours	indicates adrenal gland, ovarian, or testicular dysfunction
17 ketogenic steroids (17-KGS)	females: 3–15 mg./24 hours males: 5–23 mg./24 hours	
total estrogens	females during menstruating years: 4–100 mcg./24 hours males and postmenopausal females: 4–25 mcg./24 hours	
amino acids	30–650 mg. for 24 hours	metabolic disorders, kidney disease

APPENDIX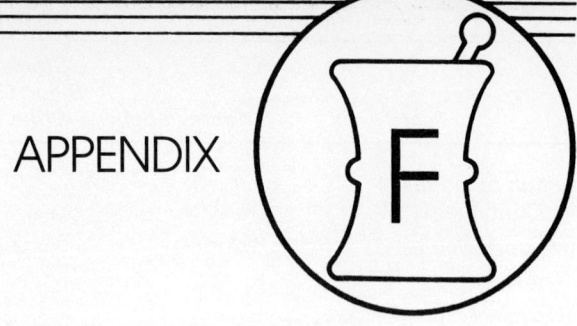

Commonly Used Diluents

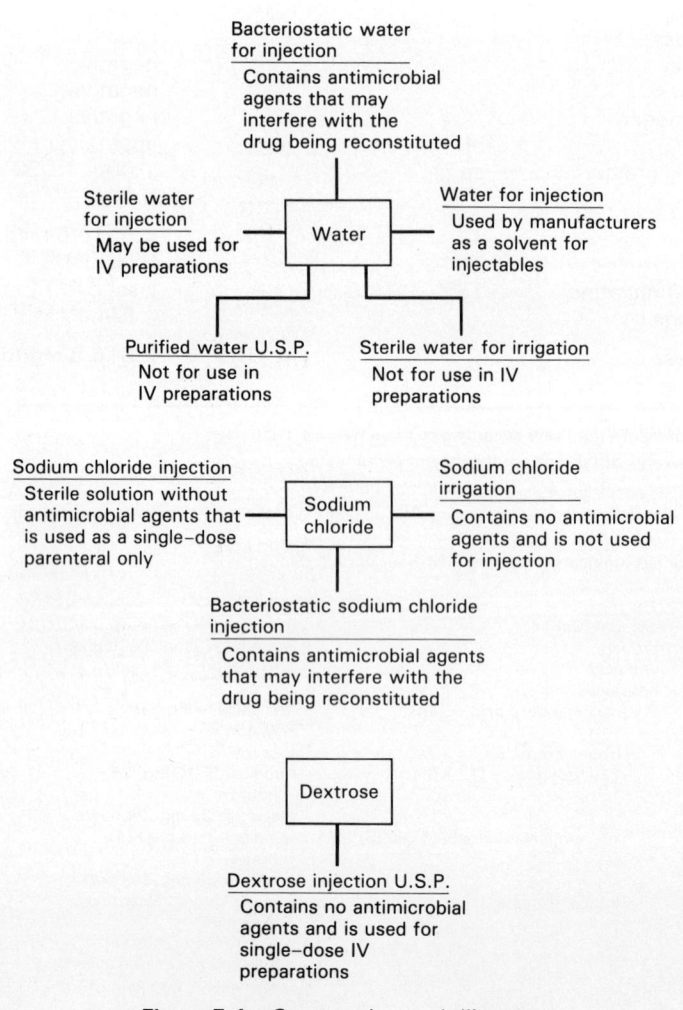

Figure F-1 Commonly used diluents.

APPENDIX G

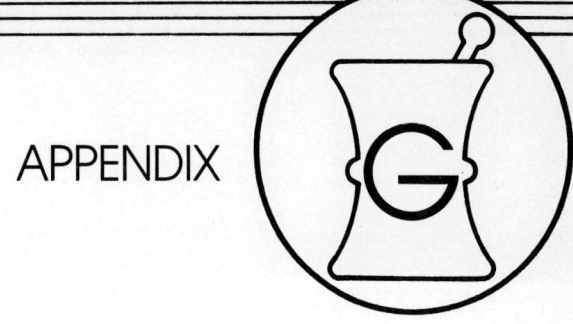

Common Vitamin Names

Vitamin	Name
Vitamin A	beta carotene
Vitamin B-6	pyridoxine
Vitamin B-1	thiamine
Vitamin B-12	cyanocobalamine (a hematinic)
Vitamin C	ascorbic acid
Vitamin D	calcifediol
	calcitriol
	dihydrotachysterol
	ergocalciferol
Vitamin E	tocopherol
Vitamin K	menadiol (K-3)
	phytonadione (K-1)
Folic acid	folate
Niacin	nicotinic acid
Niacinamide	nicotinamide (B-3)
Vitamin B-5	pantothenic acid
Vitamin B-2	riboflavin

Notes: Folic acid, niacin, niacinamide, pantothenic acid, and riboflavin are part of the B-complex vitamins. Vitamins A, D, E, and K are fat soluble vitamins. Vitamin C and the B-complex vitamins are water soluble.

APPENDIX H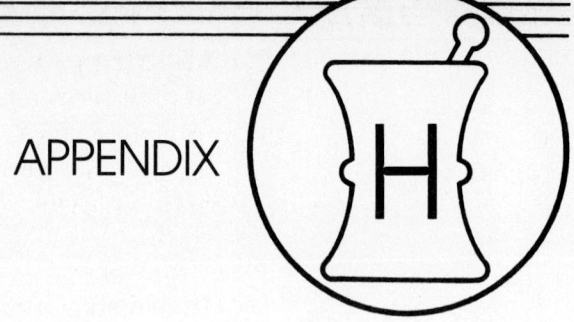

Drugs New and Coming Through

Keeping up when technology moves ahead rapidly is demanding and necessary. The following drugs are either new or in a drug testing phase. You should keep current and follow these and other drugs in a dynamically changing pharmacy environment.

Amiprilose (THERFECTIN) is an antiarthritic drug formulated from a carbohydrate prototype.

Ciprofloxacin (CIPRO) and **norfloxacin (NOROXIN)** are two antibacterial drugs of the quinolone drug class. Ciprofloxacin is indicated for acute infections of the lower respiratory tract, urinary tract, integumentary system, bones, joints, and infectious diarrhea, while norfloxacin is currently indicated for urinary tract infections only.

Ipratropium bromide (ATROVENT) is a bronchodilator which works differently than the traditional bronchodilators. Ipratropium bromide is indicated for the treatment of chronic obstructive pulmonary disease (COPD).

Lovastatin (MEVACOR), the first of a new class of cholesterol-lowering drugs, is a "reductase inhibitor" indicated for patients who have not responded successfully to nonpharmacologic measures.

Pentamidine (PENTAM 300) has been used as an inhalant for Pneumocystis carinii pneumonia (PCP) in patients with acquired immunodeficiency syndrome (AIDS). Pentamidine is FDA-approved and available in a parenteral solution dosage form.

Fluconazole is a triazole agent focusing on cryptococcosis (cryptococcal meningitis) in AIDS patients.

Zidovudine or **azidothymidine (RETROVIR, AZT)** is a virus inhibitor indicated for management in AIDS patients or AIDS related complex (ARC) patients with human immunodeficiency virus (HIV).

Other drugs which may be promising therapy for AIDS patients include:

ansamycin (RIFABUTIN)
antimonytungstate
trisodium phosphonoformate
imuthiol

Glossary

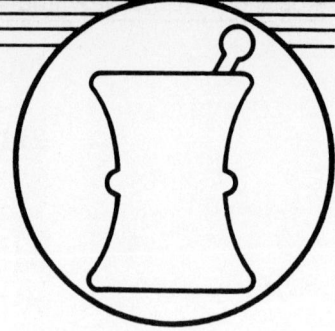

ANS acronym for autonomic nervous system
Admixture preparation of an intravenous fluid containing a drug or electrolyte which has been added to a larger volume solution
Anatomy refers to the body parts, structure, and systems
Antibiotic drug used to treat infection caused by bacteria, virus, fungus, and other living microscopic organisms
Antilipemics cholesterol-reducing agents
Aseptic pertaining to the methods used to minimize infiltration of pyrogenic and pathogenic contamination
Automatic stop order (ASO) refers to a time limit for the use of specific drugs in the hospital setting
Bolus one mass injection as opposed to a continuous administration over a period of time
Bradycardia abnormally slow heart rate
CNS acronym for central nervous system
Catecholamines body biochemicals; serotonin, dopamine, norepinephrine, and epinephrine
Catheter a hollow tube
Cell membrane covering which surrounds each cell; permits only selected substances to pass through
Central venous system vascular system directly entering and leaving the heart
Cerumen ear wax
Chronotropic referring to the effect on heart rate
Collagen diseases a collective term which refers to disorders affect-

ing the body's connective tissue; includes arthritis, rheumatism, scleroderma, and systemic lupus erythematosus (SLE)

Compromised term used to indicate a patient with a dysfunction
Coomb's test a laboratory test used to determine hemolytic anemia
Cytology study of cell structure and function
Cytoplasm living substance in a cell which surrounds the nucleus
DEA acronym for the Drug Enforcement Agency
DNA acronym for desoxyribonucleic acid; an essential part of the gene makeup
Dehydration a condition characterized by excessive water loss
Diffusion process by which molecules disperse themselves equally throughout an available space
Digitalization individual adjustment of digoxin to achieve an effective dosage
Diluent fluid used to dissolve drugs in solid form
Diuresis urination
Drip slow administration of an intravenous fluid dropwise
Endocrine glands organs which pass their secretions directly into the blood system
Epilepsy a disorder characterized by seizures
Equilibrium a state of equality
Exacerbate a worsening condition
Exocrine glands organs which secrete substances via ducts
Filtration process by which larger sized substances are strained out of liquids
Formulary a list of drugs acceptable for dispensing; usually found in the hospital
Glossitis inflammation of the tongue
Half-life the time it takes for one-half of the drug to be metabolized
Homeostasis a state of physiologic equilibrium
Hormones chemical substances produced by the body which elicit responses with only minute amounts
Hypercalcemia state in which the body's calcium level is abnormally high
Hyperkalemia state in which the body's potassium level is abnormally high
Hypermagnesemia state in which the body's magnesium level is abnormally high
Hypernatremia an above-normal level of serum sodium
Hypertension high blood pressure
Hypertonic a salt solution with a concentration greater than 0.9%
Hypocalcemia state in which the body's calcium level is very low
Hypokalemia state in which the body's potassium level is very low
Hypomagnesemia state in which the body's magnesium level is very low
Hyponatremia a below-normal level of serum sodium
Hypotonic a salt solution with a concentration less than 0.9%
Icterus jaundice; yellow complexion

Inflammation a condition characterized by redness, heat and swelling
Infusion a drug administered into the body by way of a vein for therapeutic purposes
Inotropic pertains to the effect on muscular contractility especially referring to the heart muscle
Integumentary pertains to skin, hair, and nails
Laminar flow hood a specialized workspace designed to prepare intravenous fluids in a pyrogen-free and pathogen-free environment
Loading dose an initial amount of drug used in a procedure to determine an effective dosage
Maintenance dose a drug dosage that provides therapeutic effect with minimal risk of toxicity
Miosis constriction of the eye's pupil
Morphogenetic pertaining to structural development
Mydriasis dilation of the eye's pupil
Nosocomial pertaining to the hospital setting as in nosocomial infections
NSAIA acronym for nonsteroidal anti-inflammatory agents
Nucleus the component of the cell responsible for all activities coordination
Osmosis a special type of diffusion which relies on a semipermeable membrane separating two solutions of unequal concentrations
PNS acronym for peripheral nervous system
PRN acronym for "pro re nata" meaning "when needed"
Palpitations pulsations or throbbing, usually referring to the beat of the heart
Paradoxical responses drug effects completely opposite to the expected effect
Parenteral pertaining to the injectable route directly or indirectly into blood vessels, outside the gastrointestinal tract
Particulate matter undissolved substances present in parenteral products
Pathogens disease-producing organisms
Peripheral pertaining to areas on the body surface
Peristalsis progressive wave motion as in the intestines
Permeability selective passage through a membrane
Photosensitivity increased sensitivity to sunlight
Physiology refers to the functions of the body's systems, responsibilities, and how it works
Piggyback term used to define the delivery of a secondary IV medication from an outside source into an existing large-volume IV solution
Posology study of drug dosages
Presents term used to indicate that a patient has a problem, found in journal case entries
Protocol a set of steps which are to be followed
Pruritus itching

Pyrogens fever-producing organisms
RNA acronym for ribonucleic acid; an essential part of the gene makeup
Rebound a paradoxical phenomenon in which a drug causes the effect opposite to the one intended
Salt sodium chloride
Script prescription
Sepsis a condition characterized by fever and caused by pyrogenic or pathogenic microorganisms or their toxins
Spasms painful muscle contractions
Sterile free of all living organisms
Steroids a group of compounds which include D vitamins, certain hormones and some man-made products
System groups of organs joined to perform a specialized function
Tachycardia abnormally fast heart rate
Titration process used to slowly build up a drug dosage to an effective or maintenance level
Tolerance a time-related reduction in drug effectiveness
Toxins poison
USP acronym for United States Pharmacopeia
Vasodilation a response representing an increasing diameter of the blood vessels

Index

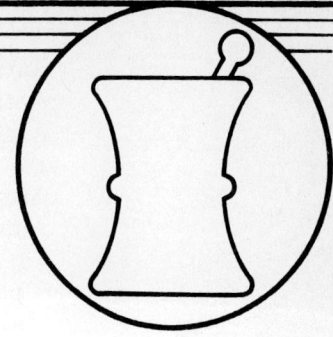

A

Acebutolol, 8, 106, 111
Acetaminophen, 48, 50, 53, 58, 70, 99
Admixture, 131
Adrenal glands:
  adrenalin (epinephrine), 63, 65, 126
  function of, 65
  noradrenalin (norepinephrine), 63, 65
Anatomy, 43
Anesthetics, 61, 70, 116
Antacids, 61
Antianginals, 106
Antiarrhythmic agents, 56, 106
Antiarthritic agents, 114–15
Antibacterial (*see* Antibiotics)
Antibiotics, 10, 22, 47, 49, 53, 56, 58, 68, 70, 116, 122 (*see also* Antineoplastics; Beta-lactams; Cephalosporins)
Anticholinergics, 51, 105
Anticoagulants, 56
Anticonvulsants, 51, 53, 114
Antidepressants, 22, 109–10
Antidiabetic agents, 66, 108, 117
Antidiarrheal agents, 61, 100
Antiemetics, 53, 61, 117
Antiflatulence medications, 61
Antifungals, 47, 53, 61, 70, 103, 116, 121–22
Antiglaucoma agents, 116
Antigout, 10, 112
Antihistamines, 22, 47, 56, 58, 61, 70, 100–101, 117, 121
Antihypercalcemic agents, 49
Antihypertensive agents, 56, 106, 110–11
Anti-infective, 101–3, 116, 120–21
Anti-inflammatory agents (*see* Nonsteroidal anti-inflammatory agents)
Antilipemics, 106
Antimalarials, 115
Antimetabolites, 104
Antimicrobials, 61
Antinauseant agents, 117
Antineoplastics, 47, 56, 61, 103–5
Antiobesity agents, 123
Antiparasitics, 103
Antiparkinson agents, 53, 119
Antiprotozoan, 70, 103
Antipyretics, 58
Antispasmodics, 61, 118–19
Antitubercular agents, 58, 103
Antitussives, 58, 119–20

Antiulcer agents, 61, 105
Antivirals, 10, 47, 103, 116, 121
Aspirin, 48, 50, 53, 58, 70, 99, 112, 115
Atropine, 51, 61, 118–19
Autonomic nervous system (ANS) (see also Nervous system)
   parasympathetic, 52
   sympathetic, 52

B

Beta-adrenergic blocking agents, 56, 106, 111
Beta-lactams, 101–2
Blood modifiers, 118
Blood pressure (BP), 55
Body systems:
   cardiovascular, 54–57
   circulatory, 54–57
   defined, 44
   digestive, 59–62
   endocrine, 62–67
   female reproductive, 69–71
   integumentary, 46–47
   male reproductive, 67–69
   muscular, 49–51
   nervous, 51–54
   pulmonary, 57–59
   respiratory, 57–59
   skeletal, 47–49
Bones, 48
   appendicular skeleton, 48–49
   axial skeleton, 48–49
   vertebral column, 48
Brompheniramine, 47, 58, 101
Bronchodilator, 58, 113

C

Calcium channel blockers, 106
Cardiovascular agents, 56, 105–7
Cardiovascular/circulatory system, 54–57
   associated disorders, 55
   components, 54
   drug classes/drugs, 56
   function/responsibility, 54
   terminology, 38
   terms and definitions, 56–57
Cell, 44
   cytoplasm, defined, 44
   membrane, defined, 44
   nucleus, defined, 44
   permeability, defined, 44

Cephalosporins, 49, 101 (see also Antibiotics)
Chelating agents, 49
Chemotherapeutic agents, 66
Chemotherapy, 103
Chlorpheniramine, 47, 58, 101
Chlorpromazine, 110, 117
Chlorpropamide, 66, 117
Cholinergic drugs, 51, 61
Cholinesterase reactivators, 51
Cimetidine, 61, 105
Clonidine, 56, 106, 111
Clorazepate, 110, 114
Clotrimazole, 47, 61, 103, 121–22
Conversions:
   apothecary, 90
   common, 88, 93
   temperature, 96
Cortisone, 49, 66, 115
Cotazyme, 61
Cytology, defined, 44
Cytotoxic chemotherapeutic agents, 70

D

Decimals, 73–78
Dermatology, 46, 120–22
Dermis, defined, 47
Desoxyribonucleic acid (DNA), 44
Desquamation, defined, 47
Dexamethasone, 53, 56, 115, 120–21
Diazepam, 110, 112, 114
Diethylstilbesterol (DES), 66, 105
Diffusion, 45
Diflunisal, 112, 115
Digestive system, 59–62
   associated disorders, 60
   components, 59
   drug classes/drugs, 60–61
   function/responsibility, 59
   terminology, 39
   terms and definitions, 61–62
Digitoxin, 56, 105
Digoxin, 7, 56, 105
Dimenhydrinate, 53, 61, 101, 117
Diphenhydramine, 47, 56, 58, 70, 101, 117, 119–21
Diuretics, 56, 61, 66, 70, 107
DNA (see Desoxyribonucleic acid)
Dosage, 8, 87
   form, 24
Drug Enforcement Administration (DEA), 18, 20–21

Drug formulary, 24
Drug levels:
  therapeutic, 72
  toxic, 72
Drug monograph, 91
Drugs:
  adverse effects, 9
  class, defined, 8
  common abbreviations, 27–33
  effects on existing disorders, 9
  effects on lab tests, 9–10
  generic names, 7
  interactions, 9
  side effects, 11–14
  trade (brand) names, 7

E

Edema, 45
Electrolyte replacements, 56, 66, 114
Endocrine system, 62–67
  associated disorders, 66
  components, 62
  drug classes/drugs, 66
  function/responsibility, 63
  terms and definitions, 67
Epidermis, defined, 47
Epinephrine (see Adrenal glands)
Equilibrium, 45
Erythromycin, 7, 47, 49, 56, 58, 103, 116, 121
Estradiol (estrogen), 65
  ethinyl, 70
Estrogen, 49, 65–66, 108 (see also Estradiol)
  combinations, 70

F

Fertility drugs, 66, 70
Festal, 61
Filtration, 45
5-fluorouracil, 47, 61, 70, 104
Furosemide, 56, 61, 66, 107

G

Gastrointestinal agents, 61, 118
Gentamicin, 116, 121
Glands (see also specific gland)
  endocrine, 63
  exocrine, 63
Glipizide, 66, 117
Glyburide, 66, 117

Gold compounds, 49, 115
Gonads:
  female hormones, 65
  function of, 65
  male hormone, 65

H

Haloperidol, 110, 117
Hemaglobin (Hgb), 56
Hematology, 54
  hematologist, 54
  vascular surgeon, 54
Histamine H_2-receptor blockers, 61
Homatropine, 116, 118
Homeostasis, 44–45
Hormones, 49, 63, 66–67, 70, 104, 107–8, 123
  adrenocorticotropic (ACTH), 64
  glucocorticoids (sugar), 63, 65, 108
  insulin, 63
  mineralocorticoids (salt), 63, 65, 107
  morphogenetic function, 63
  sex, 66, 108
  steroids, 63
  thyroid (thyroxine), 63
Hydrochlorothiazide, 7, 56, 66, 70, 107
Hydrocortisone, 47, 49, 51, 61, 66, 78, 115, 120–21
Hydroxyzine, 47, 101, 110, 117
Hypertension, 10
Hypoglycemic agents (see Antidiabetic agents)
Hypotensive agents (see Antihypertensive agents)

I

Ibuprofen, 48–49, 51, 70, 112, 115
Ilozyme, 61
Immunosuppressive drugs, 49, 51, 115
Indomethacin, 112, 115
Integumentary system, 46–47
  associated disorders, 46–47
  components, 46
  drug classes/drugs, 47
  function/responsibility, 46
  terminology, 40
  terms and definitions, 47
Intradermal, defined, 47
Intravenous hardware, 137

Intravenous therapy:
  anatomy and physiology, 127–31
  therapeutic tools, 131–36
Iron preparations, 56

K

Keratin, defined, 47

L

Laminar flow hood, 135
Laxatives, 61, 108–9
Lesions:
  macule, 47
  nodule, 47
  papule, 47
  pustule, 47
  telangiectasia, 47
  vesicle, 47
  wheal, 47
Levothyroxine, 66, 92
Loperamide, 61, 100, 113
Lorazepam, 110, 114

M

Macule, defined, 47
Measures (*see* Weights and measures)
Medical terminology:
  prefix, 35, 37–38
  root, 35
    cardiovascular system, 38
    digestive system, 39
    genitourinary system, 39
    integumentary system, 40
    musculo-skeletal system, 40
    nervous system, 40
    respiratory system, 41
    sense organs, 41
  suffix, 35
    diagnostic, 35, 41
    operative, 35, 42
    symptomatic, 35, 42
Medroxyprogesterone, 70, 105
Methotrexate, 47, 51, 70, 104
Miconazole, 47, 103, 121–22
Minerals, 62, 114
Minimum inhibitory concentration (MIC), 92
Muscle relaxants, 49–50, 112–13

Muscles:
  involuntary, 50
  voluntary, 50
Muscular system, 49–51
  associated disorders, 50
  components, 50
  drug classes/drugs, 50–51
  function/responsibility, 50
  terminology, 40
  terms and definitions, 51
Myology, 49

N

Naproxen, 112, 115
Narcotics, 48, 53, 99
Nerve blocking agents, 49, 51
Nervous system, 51–54
  associated disorders, 53
  autonomic (ANS), 51–52
  central (CNS), 51
  components, 51
  drug classes/drugs, 53
  effectors, 52
  function/responsibility, 51
  peripheral (PNS), 51
  receptors, 52
  somatic (SNS), 52
  synapses, 52–53
  terminology, 40
  terms and definitions, 54
Nitroglycerin, 7, 56, 73, 91, 106
Nodule, defined, 47
Nonsalicylates, 48
Nonsteroidal anti-inflammatory agents (NSAIA), 22, 49, 51, 70, 99–100, 111–12, 115–16, 120–21
Nonsteroidal estrogen antagonist, 70
NSAIA (*see* Nonsteroidal anti-inflammatory agents)
Nutritional agents, 49, 51
  supplements, 113–14

O

Oil glands (*see* Sebaceous)
Ophthalmic, 115–16
  diagnostic agents, 116
  lubricant, 116
Osmosis, 45
Osteology, 47

Otic agents, 120
   decongestant, 120

P

Pancreas:
   function of, 64
   glucagon, 64
   insulin, 63–64
   tolazamide, 63
   tolbutamide, 63
Pancreatic supplements, 61
Papavarine, 56, 106
Papule, defined, 47
Parathyroid gland:
   function of, 64
   hormone, 64
Parenteral routes, 126–27, 129
Partial parenteral nutrition, 133–35
Penicillin, 47, 49, 56, 58, 68, 70, 102 (*see also* Beta-lactams)
Percentage, 78–83
   concentration, defined, 93
Pharmaceutical abbreviations, 25–26
Pharmaceutical symbols, 27
Phenobarbital, 53, 70, 73, 110, 114
Phenothiazine, 61, 100
Phenylbutazone, 49, 51, 112, 115
Phenylephrine, 58, 78, 110, 120
Phenytoin, 51, 53, 114
Physician's Desk Reference, 5, 92
Physician's Order, 15, 23–24
Physiology:
   defined, 43–44
   processes, 45 (*see also* Diffusion; Filtration; Osmosis)
Piroxicam, 112, 115
Pituitary:
   function of, 64
   hormones, 64, 108
Plasma, defined, 55
Prednisolone, 104, 115, 120
Prednisone, 47, 49, 51, 53, 61, 66, 70, 104, 115
Prescription, 15–23
   elements, 18
   labels, 22
      "strip," 23
   problems, 20
   Rx, 18
   serial number, 22
PRN, defined, 25

Probenecid, 49, 112
Procainamide, 56, 106
Prochlorperazine, 61, 101, 110, 117
Progesterone, 65, 108
Promethazine, 101, 110, 117
Propantheline, 105, 119
Propoxyphene, 48, 53, 100
Propranolol, 56, 106
Psychotherapeutic agents, 109–10
Pustule, defined, 47

Q

Quinidine, 56, 106

R

Ranitidine, 61, 105
Ratio and proportion, 84–86
Reference guides, 5–6
Reproductive system:
   female, 69–71
   male, 67–69
Reserpine, 56, 111
Respiratory/pulmonary system, 57–59
   associated disorders, 58
   components, 57
   drug classes/drugs, 58
   function/responsibility, 57
   terminology, 41
   terms and definitions, 58–59
Ribonucleic acid (RNA), 44
RNA (*see* Ribonucleic acid)
Route of administration, 22
Rx, defined, 18 (*see also* Prescription)

S

Salicylates, 48, 99
Script (*see* Prescription)
Sebaceous, 46
   defined, 47
"Secundem artem," 3
Sedatives, 53, 61, 70, 110
Skeletal system, 47–49
   associated disorders, 48
   components, 48
   drug classes/drugs, 48–49
   function/responsibility, 48
   terminology, 40
   terms and definitions, 49
Sodium chloride, 45

Sphygmomanometer, 55
Spine (see Vertebrae)
Spironolactone, 56, 61, 107
Steroids, 47, 49, 51, 56, 58, 61, 63, 66, 70, 115
Stimulants, 53, 110
Subcutaneous, 47
Sucralfate, 61, 105
Sulfonamides, 68, 102
Sulindac, 112, 115
Symbols, common, 89
Sympathomimetics, 56, 113

T

Tamoxifen, 70, 105
Telangiectasia, defined, 47
Temazepam, 110
Tetracycline, 7, 47, 53, 56, 58, 61, 68, 70, 102, 116, 121
Thymus gland, function of, 65
Thyroid agents, 66
Thyroid extract, 66, 73
Thyroid gland:
   function of, 64
   hormones, 64, 108
Tissues:
   blood, 44
   connective, 44
   epithelial, 44
   formation of, 44
   muscle, 44
   nerve, 44
Tolazamide, 66, 117
Tolbutamide, 66, 117
Tolmetin, 112, 115
Total parenteral nutrition (TPN), 134
   electrolyte additives, 134
   elements of, 135
   solutions, 132–33
Tranquilizers, 22, 47, 53, 61, 70
Triamcinolone, 47, 121

U

Uricosuric agents, 49
Urinary agents, 119
U.S. Pharmacopeia, 90

V

Vaginal agents, 122–23
Vasoconstrictors, 58
Vasodilators, 56, 106
Vasopressin (Pitressin), 64, 66
Vasopressors, 56
Vertebrae (spine), 48
Vesicle, defined, 47
Viokase, 61
Vitamin B-12 preparations, 56, 129
Vitamin K preparations, 56, 129
Vitamins, 56, 113, 128–29
   defined, 62
   therapy, 66

W

Weights and measures:
   apothecary system, 87–89
      concentrations, 96
      conversions, 90
   avoirdupois, 87–88
   common equivalents, 88–89
      fluid, 93
      linear, 93
      weight, 93
   household, 87–88
   metric, 87–88, 90
      concentrations, 96
   volume to volume, 95
   weight to volume, 94
   weight to weight, 94
Wheal, defined, 47